THE BUSY EXECUTIVE'S GUIDE TO TOTAL FITNESS

ADELE PACE, M.D.
with
MARIA JONES

PRENTICE HALL
Englewood Cliffs, New Jersey 07632

Prentice-Hall International, Inc., *London*
Prentice-Hall of Australia Pty., Ltd., *Sydney*
Prentice-Hall Canada, Inc., *Toronto*
Prentice-Hall Hispanoamericana, S.A., *Mexico*
Prentice-Hall of India Private Ltd., *New Delhi*
Prentice-Hall of Japan, Inc., *Tokyo*
Prentice-Hall of Southeast Asia Pte., Ltd., *Singapore*
Editora Prentice-Hall do Brasil, Ltda., *Rio de Janeiro*

This book is a reference work based on research by the author.
The opinions expressed herein are not necessarily those of or
endorsed by the publisher. The directions stated in this book are
in no way to be considered as a substitute for consultation with
a duly licensed doctor.

10 9 8 7 6 5 4 3 2 1

Library of Congress Cataloging-in-Publication Data

Pace, Adele.
    The busy executive's guide to total fitness / Adele Pace, with
Maria Jones.
        p.   cm.
    Includes index.
    ISBN 0-13-310855-4
    1. Executives—Health programs.   2. Executives—Physical training.
I. Jones, Maria.   II. Title.
RA777.65.P33   1995
613.7—dc20   95-10603
                                                                CIP

ISBN 0-13-310855-4

PRENTICE HALL
Career and Personal Development
Englewood Cliffs, NJ 07632
A Simon & Schuster Company

Printed in the United States of America

CONTENTS

• CHAPTER 3 •
CREATING TIME FOR FITNESS—41

• CHAPTER 4 •
CHOOSING YOUR EXERCISE—55

• CHAPTER 5 •
DOING YOUR EXERCISE—77

• CHAPTER 6 •
FLEXING YOUR MUSCLES—93

• CHAPTER 7 •
EXERCISING OPTIONS—111

• CHAPTER 8 •
TAKE-HOME FITNESS—131

• CHAPTER 9 •
MANAGING YOUR PROGRESS—151

• CHAPTER 10 •

PREVENTING INJURIES—167

• CHAPTER 11 •

BALANCING YOUR NUTRITION—189

• CHAPTER 12 •

EVERYDAY EATING STRATEGIES—205

• CHAPTER 16 •
A WOMAN'S PROGRAM—275

• CHAPTER 17 •
TOTAL FITNESS—295

INDEX—303

PREFACE

In my midtwenties, a time when I was supposedly blessed with the vigor and glow of youth, I was 20 pounds overweight, couldn't run a half of a block, and didn't even entertain the thought of doing one push-up. I had no vigor, no glow. But something told me there was more to life than just being a physical failure.

In the years that followed I became a board-certified psychiatrist, studied and experimented with all aspects of fitness, joined the Medical Corps of the Army Reserve, and graduated as a Master Fitness Trainer from its national physical fitness school. I worked diligently and made mistakes along the way—the ridiculous diets, the unnecessary injuries—but always I kept my mind open, listening to the experiences of others and learning from my own.

Though they won't admit it, most executives harbor deep self-doubts about their ability to become fit. They think being fit is for the professional athlete, physically gifted, and monetarily motivated. But if this were true, no one would make it through Army basic training. In the Army, a competent instructor leads you through everything you need to learn. You are never asked if you can do it; the Army assumes that you can—whether *you* think so or not. The result: you find yourself accomplishing things that you never thought you were capable of. It's an astonishingly effective method of training.

As a psychiatrist it's my business to understand a person's limitations and potential. As a Master Fitness Trainer I know how to lead you to total fitness. Helping others by sharing my knowledge and experience is a deep desire of mine; it is the vigor and the glow I now seek. Everyone is athletically gifted enough to become totally fit. Believe in yourself and follow my lead. You will get there.

INTRODUCTION

Today's business world challenges executives more than ever. Global competition and scarce resources force business leaders to reexamine their organization's structure and their management style, to reach into their executive toolboxes for such techniques as benchmarking and reengineering, and to ask themselves what more they can do to gain a competitive edge.

But in the push for more creativity and higher productivity, executives are reaching within only to realize a frustrating truth: they are not trained to manage their most valuable asset—their true potential. Everyone has immense potential. What makes the difference between the accomplishments of two people is not how much potential they have—within the executive ranks it's quite similar—it's how much of their potential they use. Look at the leaders of the business world. Do they have some special gift? Are they geniuses or superpeople? No; they are people who merely use more of their potential.

How well you use your potential depends on your physical and emotional health. The body and the mind must be both in top shape and in concert with each other. No sedentary citizen ever reaches his potential or even comes close to it; the sheer infirmity of his physical condition prevents it. Nor can the well-conditioned athlete beat the competition if his mind is mired in wasteful distractions.

Let's start with your physical condition. Are you in better shape than the general population because you exercise more? A recently published public health report says no. Focusing on a group of highly paid, well-educated, self-motivated people who had the behavior skills to plan an exercise program, in other words today's executive, the researchers found that 50 percent of those who started an exercise program quit it within six months. Yet when asked how they felt about exercise, these same people said that they wished they did more of it. They just didn't know how to go about it.

Obviously the solution to fitness success is something not found in the corporate environment; your peers and subordinates don't have it. Nor do your leaders. What you need is the right information and the guidance to show you how to use that information in your daily life.

The Busy Executive's Guide to Total Fitness is tailored specifically for the business executive. Other books aim at everyone, selling "pain-for-gain" exercise programs or fad diets that fail. And fail everyone does. This is a book about success. It's about exercising your heart, about strengthening and toning your muscles, about eating to stay young, about thriving under a barrage of stress, and above all, about how you look at yourself and the world around you.

Notice that the last two topics deal with the mental aspects of fitness. Stress is a fact of life, and it isn't going to go away; executives must become more resilient to it. As for your attitude, the lens through which you look at the world, it is the most important determinant of success, coloring all that you experience in your fitness program. A positive attitude illuminates new horizons. A negative attitude darkens every aspect of your life.

Few fitness programs touch on attitude and even fewer aim at all aspects of fitness. Most programs aim at one aspect of fitness, for example, aerobic exercise, which is better than nothing. But this approach won't make you totally fit. Today's executive needs balance and strength in all areas of his responsibility. The same goes for your fitness. Working on one aspect of fitness is only a beginning. From there you move into other areas, not haphazardly but carefully, perhaps changing your diet or building your strength. You choose the order. That's an important point. Everyone is different, with different needs; therefore no fitness program should impose an order on you. What this program does is introduce you to each aspect of fitness by giving you insightful information about the needs and responses of your body. Then you're shown how to get started and move forward. Each move will be a milestone, each goal reached a triumph. Ultimately you'll be *looking* for new ways to improve your fitness—the joy is as much in the journey as it is in reaching the goal.

Armed with a balanced approach, convinced that it will empower you in the business world, you are truly ready to start a program. But how can you fit it into an impossibly packed schedule? Your career and family already take up all your time and energy. Relax—and take another look, first through this book and then through your life. Is there a way to create more time? Yes. Can you pursue fitness in a business environment that is a minefield of roadblocks, from busy seasons, frequent travel, and inflexible schedules to inevitable crises and long hours? Yes. Any guide to total fitness must show you how to hurdle these roadblocks, and *The Busy Executive's Guide to Total Fitness* does.

With a step-by-step approach, you'll build a firm foundation—then a skyscraper on top of it. There are no gimmicks, no quick fixes—these don't exist. But miracles do, and they will happen within you.

Unlike executives of the past, you want and need more. You want the unbeatable feeling of being in control of your body and mind, of knowing that you can handle any personal and business crisis that comes your way, benefits only total fitness can give you.

The human body is a marvelous organism. Given the right care, it can do things you never dreamed possible, like build skyscrapers. Every executive needs a healthy body and alert mind. It's not easy to endure stress-filled workdays week after week, year after year. You need something more: the ultimate competitive edge God meant you to have. Let this total fitness program help you gain it. Propel yourself to a higher level of performance. Build that skyscraper. Don't shortchange yourself by putting this book down without reading it.

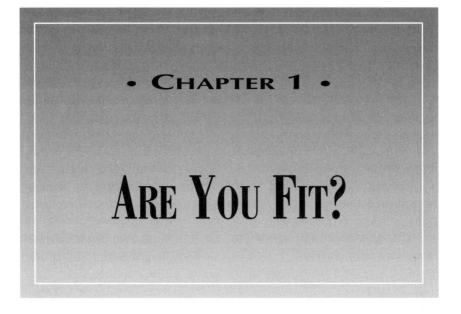

ARE YOU FIT?

It was late September 1983 and I was about to become a runner. I felt great—filled with energy and confidence as I bounded out the door for my first 20-minute run. It was a confidence born of constant activity: walking 15 blocks from Manhattan's Penn Station to First Avenue and back five days a week and housecleaning and gardening on weekends. Surely I was fit enough to run a few blocks. But I was wrong. As I neared the end of the first block, my lungs began to burn with every inadequate breath and the legs that were supposed to carry me another 19 minutes began to drag with every stride. I felt ill.

Of course I wasn't ill, but the body I had deemed fit wasn't able to run for 20 minutes either. What I learned during that first run was that I didn't know what being fit meant. Nor did I know how to get that way. Like so many of my colleagues at the time, I thought youth, slimness, and moderate activity made me fit. To learn otherwise was a painful lesson—both physically and psychologically. It was also a blessing.

That first run woke me up. From it I learned I had to take a more specific approach to fitness: commit myself to a specific activity and gradually acclimate my body to it. Today I am fit by any standards. But it wasn't an easy journey.

On the way I had to overcome a chronic knee injury—another painful experience which granted a blessing. It forced me to investigate other exercises: cross-country skiing to strengthen my legs; weight lifting to strengthen my upper body; stretching to improve my flexibility and prevent other injuries. A whole world opened up.

Eventually I was able to run again, expanding my exercise horizon still further. But demons still haunted me, and cutthroat hospital politics, combined with an unmanageable work load, drove me to explore ways of improving my resilience against stress. Exercise is a stress reducer itself. I hate to think what navigating that period of my life would have been like without it.

Even now my journey to fitness isn't over. Every year I continue to change mentally and physically, to learn more about the miracle of fitness, and to see more proof that the world desperately needs it. My discovery of fitness was haphazard, guided by trial and error. Yours won't be.

COMMITTING YOURSELF TO A FITNESS LIFESTYLE

Perhaps you embarked on a similar journey only to become discouraged or never bothered with fitness in the first place—it was for health nuts. Or you had other concerns that seemed more pressing. Whatever your reason for being unfit, it's not good enough. Health institutions, government agencies, and private industry agree. In a joint statement the American College of Sports Medicine (ACSM) and the Centers for Disease Control described America's unfitness as an "epidemic of inactivity." It's an epidemic that kills.

Don't be a victim of this epidemic. By committing yourself to a program of total fitness, you step to the forefront of a movement certain to gain momentum and get a running start at changing yourself into a more productive person, who gets the most out of all areas of life. It's a proven success formula. Some of the most accomplished people in this country have used it to attain success without sacrificing their health.

Yet many more people have abandoned it, compiling a dropout rate so shocking that health experts began to study the problem in depth. After dividing the pursuit of fitness into two segments, adoption and adherence, they determined what factors lead to success in each. What they found out was surprising.

Whether or not a person adopted a fitness program was governed by his knowledge of health and exercise. Knowledge is a motivator, as well as a provider of facts. Without it, designing and launching a fitness program would be difficult, if not dangerous. What keeps people in the dark is impatience. They don't take the time to learn about their bodies, look into different exercises, or ask other exercisers for advice. Instead they rush into a program and fail.

Adherence, on the other hand, depended on the ability of people to overcome the numerous roadblocks that hindered their efforts. Of these, travel, injuries, and time constraints were the most notorious. No doubt these plague you. But with the proper guidance, you can handle any of them and move on to success. Knowledge and guidance are the secrets to becoming fit.

WHAT IS FITNESS?

Still, the word "fit" is a vague concept. What exactly does it mean? I'll start by telling you what it doesn't mean: fitness is not the absence of illness or disease. If that were true, anyone who seldom saw a doctor would be considered fit even though like myself years ago he could hardly run a block. Conversely, a person seriously ill with cancer can be fit. In fact, fitness improves your chances in battling any disease.

What then is fitness? Total fitness is an integrated state of body and mind. What affects you physically will affect you emotionally; likewise, what affects you emotionally will affect you physically. A severely depressed person, for example, shuffles slowly, head bowed, shoulders slumped—a body seemingly devoid of energy. His body reflects his mood. But it's not a one-way street; the mind also responds to the body. Having your movements restricted for even less than a day would make you feel downcast or depressed.

The same is true when your body is weak and inflexible. Recognizing this condition your brain sets up a parallel mind-set—one that won't possess the spontaneity or creativity your mind is capable of. Equally important is that positive changes in your physical condition improve your emotional state, just as positive emotions improve your physical condition. The mind and body are one.

For the sake of clarity, however, I will discuss fitness by separating the body and mind, and by dividing each of those categories into subcategories. Most people oversimplify fitness—it's only a good heart or strong muscles—thereby missing one or more of the physical components and both of the mental ones. To be physically fit, you must have all three components: cardiovascular endurance, muscular fitness, and a good nutritional status. To be mentally fit, you must be resilient to stress and have a healthy attitude. The second mental component, a healthy attitude, the most powerful component in its ability to influence all aspects of your life, again brings us back to the connection between physical and mental fitness—that the body and mind constantly exchange cues from each other.

Cardiovascular Endurance Comes from Exercise

Cardio endurance, the first component of physical fitness, is the ability of your heart, lungs, and blood vessels to supply your body, especially your working muscles, with oxygen. Though each of these organs benefits from conditioning, the heart and blood vessels improve the most. But why don't the lungs? Aren't they what make you gasp for air during exercise? The answer is not really. As an unfit person exercises, his muscles quickly run out of oxygen. Needing more to continue, the muscles summon the brain, which reacts by commanding the heart to beat faster and the lungs to breathe harder. The lack of oxygen, however, is not because of the lungs' inability to take in enough—they usually can—but because the heart and blood vessels cannot get this oxygen to the muscles. Team up the same unfit lungs with a well-conditioned heart and blood vessel network, and you would suffer little or no breathlessness.

But people are far more aware of their labored breathing than their rapid heart rate. That's why you see the oxygen charade during sporting events. At football games, players on the sidelines routinely place oxygen masks over their faces, as if more of this miracle gas can improve their performance. It can't. Trainers and team doctors, of course, know this. The players, however, don't. They think it helps, a belief that may be powerful enough to improve their performance, but not their lungs.

Mind games aside, the best way to banish shortness of breath is to condition your heart and blood vessels with exercise. As the heart muscle becomes stronger, it enlarges slightly, also expanding its network of blood vessels. This enables the heart to receive a larger blood supply so it too can get more oxygen during periods of heavy work. Now it can pump more blood with each beat.

More heart muscle isn't always an indication of good health. When the heart enlarges without building extra blood vessels, as in hypertrophic cardiomyopathy, it's vulnerable to irregular beats. Basketball player Hank Gathers died from this. Far more people die because of clogged blood vessels to the heart, which cut off its blood supply, thereby depriving it of oxygen. A muscle deprived of oxygen dies. Hence the part of the heart denied oxygen dies, and if it's a large enough area, the heart attack victim dies. Survivors of heart attacks are on notice: more of their heart muscle can die at any time. Clogging of blood vessels doesn't happen selectively—it happens everywhere. The prescription here is exercise. It gently conditions the heart, installing more blood vessels throughout it. Then if an obstruction occurs, there will be other blood vessels to deliver oxygen to the stricken area. Had exercising been the policy all along, the heart attack may never have happened.

Looking at the blood vessels throughout the body, we see a similar reaction to exercise. In regularly exercised muscles, not only are more blood vessels installed, but the existing ones become more elastic. Vessel elasticity is an important quality. Without it a blood vessel could not expand to let extra blood through, causing the blood pressure to rise as the heart works harder pushing. It's the difference between the same volume of water flowing through a thin plastic hose and an expandable rubber hose. Ultimately, the water pressure could burst the plastic hose. High blood pressure patients live with this threat, along with many other debilitating side effects of their disease. Again the prescription is exercise. In fact, for the cardiovascular system, the prescription is always exercise, whether you are healthy or ill.

Muscular Fitness Is Strength, Endurance, and Flexibility

Muscular fitness is the second component in the equation of total physical fitness. Consisting of three subcategories—muscle strength, muscle endurance, and muscle flexibility—it focuses on body movement. The most familiar category is muscle strength, which is the maximum force generated by a contracting muscle as measured by the maximum amount of weight you can lift only once. That is once, not two or three times. If you can lift a weight twice, you can probably lift a heavier weight once. But strictly this is a *measure* of your strength. Rarely do you exercise this way. Though strength-gaining exercises do require you to lift heavy weights, you should be able to lift them between three and ten times. By lifting such weights you stress your muscles. It's a positive stress. Muscles respond to it by building more white or "fast-twitch" muscle fiber, the generator of peak force. These fibers, however, cannot use much oxygen. Becoming exhausted too quickly, they can't maintain the effort, and therefore don't have time to use that much extra. It's an effort best described as "all or nothing."

With oxygen use relatively low—more is used only during short bursts of exercise—the heart doesn't benefit. Still, muscle strength is important. The forces generated by strong contracting muscles strengthen the bones they are attached to, making weight lifting, also called resistance exercises, an excellent defense against osteoporosis, a disease that thins or weakens the bones. Strong muscles also guard against injury. Whenever there is a sudden force or impact on the body, the difference between a bruise and a broken bone, torn muscle, ripped tendon, torn ligament, or dislocation may be the strength of the surrounding muscles. Strong muscles not only make your life easier; they make it safer.

The next category of muscular fitness is endurance. Controlled by red or "slow-twitch" fiber, endurance is the ability of a muscle to contract repeatedly for a sustained period. This is not strength; a muscle with only endurance won't be able to lift heavy objects. Rather, it is a persistence typical of slow-twitch fiber. To build this fiber, you exercise less intensely: instead of lifting heavy weights, say, 6 times, you lift lighter weights 15 to 25 times. Or you run or bike or cross-country ski.

These activities your heart likes because they are continuous in their demand for extra oxygen and the heart must keep working hard to provide it—exactly what it needs to stay healthy. But the muscles demanding oxygen must be large. Small muscle groups, by themselves, can't tax the heart enough to make it stronger, another reason why weight lifting, which usually works small groups, does not benefit it. Look at all endurance sports. Running, biking, rowing—these work the lower body, where the largest muscle groups are located. And as an added bonus, endurance also protects you from injury.

Flexibility is the final component of muscular fitness. Truly the Rodney Dangerfield of its genre, it gets no respect—many people dismiss it as sort of double-jointedness, an innate ability bestowed upon athletes. It isn't. It is the elasticity of muscles and tendons attained through regular stretching. In professional and amateur sports flexibility is crucial. It ensures athletes a wide range of motion, which even more than strength and endurance, protects them from injury. In fact, there are flexibility coaches because a pulled muscle can lose a championship and a torn tendon can forfeit a title. The bottom line for athletes is dollars—perhaps millions. But what's in it for you? An inactive person who doesn't expose himself to the rigors of exercise, and its potential for injury, is actually hurt far more frequently and severely than a person who is fit and flexible. As a flexible person you can assume more postures and perform more movements. This affects how you feel, both physically and emotionally. Your bottom line—better quality of life.

You Are What You Eat

The third physical component of fitness is nutrition status, bringing to life the well-known phrase, "You are what you eat." Becoming what you eat sounds more humorous than frightening. Too many visits to junk-food land won't turn you into a donut, french fry, or frankfurter. Unfortunately, it can do worse. What you eat affects how you look, feel, act, and even think. Considering how bad a poor diet can make you feel, how bleakly it can color your entire life, I would rather turn into a donut—at least I'd have eternal police protection, and plenty of caffeine.

Taking that phrase seriously is one thing; applying it to yourself is another. Most people don't. Part of the problem is denial: you don't really eat that way. Another part is lack of awareness. When asked to recall what they ate during one day, people who sincerely tried to remember, couldn't. They thought they ate less, and when they did remember, they didn't know what was actually in the food or how it affected their health. An egg and sausage biscuit, for example, may sound wholesome, but when eaten regularly it saturates your diet—and, of course, your body—with fat. Now you may think you don't eat much junk food and therefore your diet isn't high in fat. But sausage biscuits along with many other popular foods contain so much fat that even when eaten in moderation, they launch the percentage of fat in your diet. A high-fat diet makes you fat. Only extremely active people escape this fate; yet they are by no means safe. That they don't gain weight is only part of the story. What they do get from fatty foods are clogged arteries, cancers, and many other maladies. For those who are not active, the downfall is more obvious.

The human body wasn't made to be fat. As man evolved, fat tissue was a mode of survival, providing energy during lean times. It was not and is not meant to cover the body constantly. Under such a burden the body simply doesn't function as well. Overweight people have less energy, a condition that depletes them mentally and fatigues them easily—even from moderate activities. In a society smitten with slimness, this does not go unnoticed. Studies have shown that overweight people get fewer promotions, which coincides with their consistently lower pay, and that women, in addition to these career complications, fare poorly in the social sphere. Fewer of them marry. Obesity is a social disease too.

The problems with many diets are not limited to excess fat. The wrong proportion of nutrients, not enough vitamins, too little fiber—these also interfere with the function of your body and mind. Then there is the how of your eating habits. Under what circumstances do you usually eat? Is there chaos—people in and out, phone calls, arguments, a TV blaring? Do you eat on the run, snack mindlessly, skip meals, binge at night? This affects your digestion and nutrient absorption. Ultimately, *you are what you eat* and that is a big part of fitness.

Building Up Your Stress Resilience

Having discussed all the physical aspects of fitness, let's look at the mental ones. First, not everyone is mentally sound: a small number of people do suffer from mental illness. That is outside the scope of this book. What is within it is the majority of people who are mentally sound, but may not be using their minds as effectively as possible. Neuropsychologists have determined that we use less than 1 percent of our brain's capacity. One percent. That's minute compared to what we expect out of the machines we build. By increasing that percentage to just 2 or 3 percent, we could double or triple our mental power. But that is a quantum gain. With much smaller gains we could increase our productivity and improve the quality of our lives.

Stress and a person's response to it depends on the individual. Executives must learn to deal with adverse events over which they have little or no control almost on a daily basis. Distinct to male executives is the vulnerability of their heart to stress and their tendency to lean on alcohol in stressful situations. Female executives must cope with the socially conflicting dual roles of professional and homemaker-mother.

Exercise—the type that builds your cardiovascular endurance—quiets your mind and relaxes your body. Morning exercise is especially effective in improving your sleep patterns, giving you better rest when you're asleep and more energy when you're awake. But exercise done at any hour not only relieves tension in an executive's busy life, it is a powerfully positive force that defends you from negative thoughts. It overpowers the emotions of anxiety and depression and can even inspire some of your most creative ideas.

Exercise cannot remove stress from your life. Nothing can. Stress simply exists, and you must accept that. But how you handle stress depends on your stress resilience. Probably you've heard of stress management, with its collection of techniques that change your behavior so that you can better cope with the stressors that bombard you daily. Some executives use these techniques as a routine part of their behavior. But they never learned them in school or at seminars. Instead, they picked them up from a parent, or learned it from a mentor, or discovered it through experimentation, noticing that certain approaches gave relief. How lucky they are. Not as lucky are many more people, who despite their success, have no such skills. For those people life is an ongoing battle; they are pounded by today's fast-paced and stressful business environment. To keep up, they use an arsenal of destructive habits and tactics that stunt their ability and dull the quality of their lives. What is so disparaging is that many of them don't even realize it. They have been tense all their lives and think it's a normal state instead of a destructive one. Or they are pessimists who think stress management won't work for them, that it is just another way for consultants to make money.

By exercising and practicing techniques specifically designed to alleviate the effects of stress, you can greatly improve your mental health, and in an era of global competition, this may be your best competitive edge.

Shaping Your Attitude for Positive Results

Why people neglect their stress resilience is a function of their attitudes, and they contort their reasoning into many stirring rationalizations to support it. Such is the power of attitude—the second component of mental fitness. But attitude affects more than your outward behavior; it affects your health as well. Take, for example, a "Type A" executive, the quintessential perfectionist, aggressive, competitive, and hard driving on every front, with a streak of hostility that's chronically inflamed by his lack of time. Here the focus is external competitiveness—him against the world—but while this may get results, they are at far too high a price. Type A-ism impairs your productivity and leaves you prone to heart disease, especially heart attacks. In the sports arena, too, external competitiveness dominates. The athlete, by concentrating on beating his opponent, drains his productivity. His physical performance suffers and he loses.

Still, not all Type A attributes are bad. Competitiveness can be good if it's directed inward. An executive with internal competitiveness always looks for ways to do his job better, to make his company better, and to make himself better, maximizing his performance. He doesn't waste time and adrenaline on beating out another executive or company. He views problems as opportunities, and when faced with a bleak situation, he manages to create success without getting angry, or critical. It's an attitude that draws out the creative powers of his brain and it shows in his accomplishments at work and at home. When you reshape the negative characteristics of your attitude into positive ones, you will live longer and healthier.

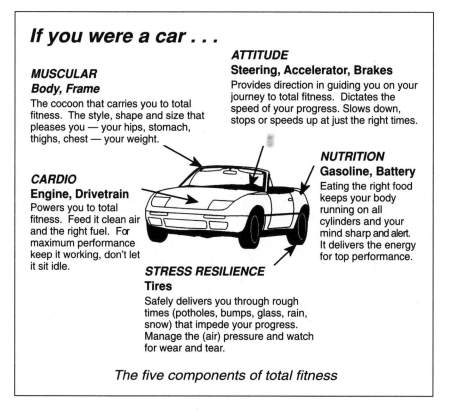

If you were a car . . .

MUSCULAR
Body, Frame
The cocoon that carries you to total fitness. The style, shape and size that pleases you — your hips, stomach, thighs, chest — your weight.

ATTITUDE
Steering, Accelerator, Brakes
Provides direction in guiding you on your journey to total fitness. Dictates the speed of your progress. Slows down, stops or speeds up at just the right times.

CARDIO
Engine, Drivetrain
Powers you to total fitness. Feed it clean air and the right fuel. For maximum performance keep it working, don't let it sit idle.

NUTRITION
Gasoline, Battery
Eating the right food keeps your body running on all cylinders and your mind sharp and alert. It delivers the energy for top performance.

STRESS RESILIENCE
Tires
Safely delivers you through rough times (potholes, bumps, glass, rain, snow) that impede your progress. Manage the (air) pressure and watch for wear and tear.

The five components of total fitness

ARE YOU FIT?

Just knowing what the components of fitness are is a huge step toward becoming fit. It motivates you by helping you to visualize what fitness is and why it is important. Another motivator is your condition. How fit are you? And where do you need the most work? Find out by answering the following fitness self-assessment questions as accurately as you can. Because the questionnaire is designed for a wide range of readers, some questions may not seem to apply to you. Answer them anyway; vague feelings usually suggest strong tendencies.

I. CARDIO

1. How often do you exercise aerobically such as jogging, cycling, swimming, or any vigorous activity for 20 minutes or more?

   a. Never
   b. Once or twice a week
   c. Three times a week
   d. More than three times a week

2. How does the exercise described in question 1 leave you feeling?

   a. Nothing—you never do it
   b. Weak and worn out
   c. Pleasantly tired
   d. Refreshed

3. How do you feel after walking up two flights of stairs?

   a. Short of breath with pain in your thighs
   b. Tired and sluggish for a while
   c. A slight leg weariness that quickly disappears
   d. No noticeable effect

4. For how long can you comfortably run at a moderate pace?

   a. Only 0–5 minutes
   b. 5–15 minutes
   c. 15–20 minutes
   d. More than 20 minutes

5. How many cigarettes do you smoke a day?

   a. More than half a pack
   b. Up to half a pack
   c. Smoked previously but not in last three years
   d. Never smoked

6. Do you go out of your way to avoid walking (such as persistently searching for close-in parking places)?

   a. Almost always
   b. Most of the time

c. Sometimes

d. Rarely

II. MUSCULAR

1. How often do you do a strength enhancing exercise such as weight lifting?

    a. Never

    b. Occasionally

    c. Once a week

    d. At least twice a week

2. How does the kind of exercise described in question 1 leave you feeling?

    a. Nothing—you never do it

    b. Shaky or weak in the muscles used

    c. No noticeable effect

    d. Pumped up, stronger

3. How many regular push-ups can you do?

a. 0–3	Male	0–2	Female
b. 4–10	Male	3–6	Female
c. 11–20	Male	7–14	Female
d. 21 +	Male	15 +	Female

4. How many sit-ups can you do (feet not held, hands over chest, 45 degrees to the floor)?

    a. 0–3

    b. 4–12

    c. 13–18

    d. 19 +

5. Can you touch your toes and maintain it for 20 seconds?

    a. No

    b. With 1–3 fingers but can't hold for 20 seconds

    c. With 1–3 fingers

    d. With 4–5 fingers

6. How often do you stretch major muscle groups?

    a. Never
    b. Rarely
    c. Twice a week
    d. Three or more times a week

III. NUTRITION

1. Are you overweight?

    a. By over 20 pounds
    b. By 10–20 pounds
    c. By 5–10 pounds
    d. No

2. How often do you eat fatty foods such as beef, bacon, sausage, pork ribs, fried foods, or foods containing large amounts of butter or cream?

    a. Daily
    b. Regularly
    c. Occasionally
    d. Rarely

3. How often do you eat fast foods?

    a. Daily other than dinner or dinner 3 or more times a week
    b. Every few days
    c. Occasionally
    d. Rarely

4. How often do you eat breakfast?

    a. Never
    b. Seldom
    c. More than half the time
    d. Daily

5. You know the nutritional content of what percent of the food you regularly eat?

    a. 0 %

  b. Up to 25 %
  c. 25–50 %
  d. 50–100 %

6. How often do you take a multiple vitamin supplement?

  a. Never
  b. Up to 3 times a week
  c. 4–5 times a week
  d. Daily

IV. STRESS

1. How often do you have more work than you can finish in a regular workday?

  a. Almost always
  b. Frequently
  c. Sometimes
  d. Infrequently

2. Are you easily annoyed, impatient, or quick to snap at others?

  a. Most of the time
  b. Frequently
  c. Occasionally
  d. Rarely

3. Are you able to relax and enjoy your vacation or recreational time?

  a. Rarely
  b. Occasionally
  c. Frequently
  d. Almost always

4. How often do you have an alcoholic drink to relax and put the day's concerns behind you?

  a. Every day
  b. Often
  c. Occasionally
  d. Rarely

5. How often do you feel responsible for situations over which you have no control?

   a. Almost always
   b. Frequently
   c. Occasionally
   d. Rarely

6. How often do you confide in or get advice from a spouse or friend?

   a. Never
   b. Infrequently
   c. Sometimes
   d. Usually

V. ATTITUDE

1. What is your response when a subordinate or coworker makes a mistake?

   a. *Anger:* it could have been avoided, should never have happened and is wasting your time and energy
   b. *Annoyance:* you decide not to delegate that responsibility again— if you want it done correctly you'll do it yourself
   c. *Disappointment:* mistakes are inevitable and can be fixed
   d. *Resolve:* you correct the person who made the mistake and take action to make the best of the situation

2. What would your response be if you heard about a competing firm's new idea, which would put them ahead of you?

   a. *Outrage:* they must have cheated in some way
   b. *Anxiety:* you must find out what it is and improve on it
   c. *Surprise:* they really outdid themselves this time
   d. *Action:* you aim at getting your own ideas to the marketplace as quickly as possible

3. How would you feel if you were handed a special project on top of all your other work?

   a. *Irate:* they are always dumping extra work on you
   b. *Worry:* where will you find the time to do it

    c. *Concern:* you decide to farm out some less important work to an assistant

    d. *Enthusiasm:* this is a real opportunity to shine even if it means a few late nights

4. What would your response be if an outside person were hired for your boss's job?

    a. *Rage:* after you repeatedly demonstrated that you were more capable than your boss

    b. *Disillusionment:* this was not part of your plan

    c. *Dismay:* you investigate other positions that may offer advancement

    d. *Surprise:* you offer the new boss your help while considering your career options

5. What would your response be if your company announced that it's opening a fitness center for employees to use?

    a. *Negative:* you don't exercise and feel it's a waste of productive work time

    b. *Disinterest:* maybe others can use the facility

    c. *Support:* you think fitness is an admirable goal to strive for and maybe you'll give it a try

    d. *Enthusiasm:* this fits in with your new resolve for fitness

6. What would your response be if a new research study revealed that a properly conducted program for total fitness will ensure success and improve the quality of your life?

    a. *Apathy:* new studies come out with erroneous findings all the time, and this is just another one

    b. *Disbelief:* success is achieved only through hard work and dedication

    c. *Curiosity:* you've been hearing a lot about fitness lately and would like to find out more

    d. *Gratification:* you felt all along that total fitness was a key to self-improvement and now a study confirms your belief

Just by answering the questions, you can get a feel for where you stand on fitness, but your questionnaire score will tell you much more. As noted on the following page each answer has a point value.

a. 0 points

b. 1 point

c. 3 points

d. 4 points

Assign the appropriate point value to your answers and add them up. Each section has a maximum of 24 points; the total questionnaire has a maximum of 120 points.

Your total score will give you an overview of your physical and emotional condition: the higher your score, the better your condition. But generalizations can be misleading. To better interpret your score, see Figure 1.1, which tells you what your score for each component means. The component scores give you a more definitive description of your condition, and are therefore more accurate than your total score.

Still, a total score is telling. One below 70 points indicates severe deficiencies in several areas or serious deficiencies in all areas. If you are in this condition, don't despair; progress from this low point is quite dramatic in the beginning. Start by forming appropriate goals. Then look forward to successes that will solidify your new habits and provide a solid foundation for continued improvement. But don't attack every component at once. Concentrate first on the ones with the lowest scores. If all your scores are comparably low, give priority to cardio fitness, followed by stress, nutrition, attitude, and muscular fitness, in that order.

A total score of 70–94 indicates either inconsistent fitness (some areas good, others poor) or adequate fitness, with all areas at a similar level. Again start in the area with the lowest score. If several or all components have a similar score, set priorities as above.

If you score above 94 points, be proud. Nevertheless, check each component of fitness for the possibility that one or more has received less attention than the others and start your improvement program there. Whatever you do, don't become complacent. In the business world today, being the most admired company is not an invitation to stand still—tomorrow can always be judged by new and different standards. Always set your sights higher. Total fitness is like business success, a moving target.

Figure 1.1   *INTERPRETATION OF FITNESS SCORES*

CARDIO

0 – 11	Seriously deficient activity level exposes you to risk of coronary and related diseases. Effects are largely reversible, but start now.
12 – 16	Some activity but not enough. Need to address some distinct problems — perhaps smoking.
17 – 19	Indicates you're in the swing of things. Be confident but not overconfident.
20 – 24	Appear to have satisfactory cardio program. May benefit from periodic intensifications. Otherwise, you're in position to make gains in other areas of fitness.

MUSCULAR

0 – 11	Problem with strength and endurance; probably inflexible. Warrants action now if no conflict with another fitness component.
12 – 16	Indicates some exercising but not enough strength building or stretching. Program needs to be "pumped up."
17 – 20	Seem to have a good strength training program. Look to refine or intensify it.
21 – 24	Powerful approach to your muscles and flexibility. Fine-tune it.

NUTRITION

0 – 12	Poor nutritional habits are harming your body. Address your problems immediately but with control not aggressiveness.
13 – 16	Indicates some good habits and some bad. Strive for a good fundamental understanding of nutrition and begin a gradual program of improvement.
17 – 20	Appear to have a few isolated problems. But if you're overweight, you probably underestimated your consumption of fat.
21 – 24	Sound nutritional habits and awareness of eating. Keep a constant vigil for ever-changing food products to maintain your status.

STRESS

0 – 12	A dark situation indicating serious problems at work or with your family. Stress management techniques are a must. A cardio program would have a positive impact.
13 – 17	A specific problem or islands of stress can harm you physically and emotionally. Address distinct concerns — perhaps alcohol.
18 – 24	Even though you may lack support at times you show a strong stress resilience. But remain aware of stressors.

ATTITUDE

0 – 12	Significant outlook difficulties. Don't expect massive transfusion of optimism overnight. Start now to toss your emotional baggage.
13 – 16	Alter your outlook or how you handle interpersonal relationships. Feel new life and increased productivity by relieving your anxieties.
17 – 24	Flexible attitude with a positive frame of mind. You're ready to launch into a total fitness program. Expect success soon.

Don't let these scores rule your attitude: too much confidence is just as bad as too little. No matter what your condition is, you're going to improve, to move forward—the right direction for anyone. Remember, the glory is in the journey.

Should You Get a Doctor's OK to Exercise?

A good score on the fitness questionnaire may not necessarily mean you are ready to start a fitness program. First observe the ACSM guidelines. A "yes" answer to any of the following questions means you should get a doctor's OK first.

1. Do you have heart trouble?

2. Do you frequently suffer from chest pains?

3. Do you often feel faint or have dizzy spells?

4. Do you have high blood pressure?

5. Do you have a bone or joint problem, such as arthritis that has been or could be aggravated by exercise?

6. Are you over age 65 and not accustomed to exercise?

7. Are you taking any prescription medications such as those for heart problems or high blood pressure?

8. Is there a good physical reason not mentioned here that could prevent you from following an activity program?

A "yes" answer does not imply that you cannot exercise; it simply tells you to see a doctor first. Total fitness is itself an excellent treatment for many of the problems just listed. People with osteoporosis, for example, are often told to lift weights. A person with joint problems (depending on their nature) could benefit from stretching and weight lifting to improve the range of motion in those joints and strengthen the surrounding muscles. For a heart patient, aerobic exercise and dietary changes are usually the prescription. And diabetes and high blood pressure respond so well to exercise that medication dosages can often be reduced.

You may be asked to take an exercise stress test. During this test, your heart is monitored while you exercise at progressively higher intensities, a procedure that spots problems early, allowing you and your doctor to plan your fitness program accordingly. The ACSM recommends a stress test for the following reasons:

1. You are over age 45.
2. You are over age 35 with at least one major *coronary risk factor* or any symptoms of cardiovascular disease. Coronary risk factors are
   a. High blood pressure
   b. Total cholesterol/HDL cholesterol index over 5
   c. Cigarette smoker
   d. Abnormal EKG
   e. Family history of coronary heart disease or other atherosclerotic disease prior to age 50
   f. Diabetes

But everyone is different. Understanding that, your doctor may suggest the test even if the ACSM criteria doesn't apply to you. If he or she does, take it; it's a worthwhile test. Besides giving you peace of mind, it tells you your maximum exercise-induced heart rate. In planning an exercise program that information gives you a tremendous advantage.

TOTAL FITNESS IS FOR ALL AGES

It's never too early or too late to become fit. Adolescence, supposedly at an age when you can get away with anything, is really a time when poor fitness begins its destructive reign. But it's not obvious, so you don't think it's happening.

Now flash ahead to middle age. Is there anything you can do about a lifetime of poor fitness? The answer is yes. Often a physical disaster, such as a heart attack, is the beginning of a rebuilding program that leaves the patient stronger—both physically and emotionally—than ever before. Or the threat of disability is the origin of a new routine. When a 58-year-old woman, stricken with disabling arthritis looked for help, she found stretching. Today at 72, she is still doing splits.

Indeed the twilight years are no exception. Elderly nursing home patients improved their strength 200 percent in three months. Their average age was 80. The ability for muscle to improve and grow stronger is as ageless as the ability to reach inside yourself and unlock hidden potential. It's a challenge. But out of it comes success—in every sphere possible.

• CHAPTER 2 •

DEVELOPING YOUR FITNESS GOALS

Have you ever wondered how hypnosis works? As one of the most enigmatic scientific procedures, it draws a wide range of reactions: from awe, as if it were magic, to cynicism, as if it were a hoax. But it's neither. By working through an unconscious state closer to alertness than to sleep, hypnosis makes you a believer. This is a two-step process. First you relax and focus your mind on one thing. Then you are told to believe something and regardless of what it is—you no longer smoke or you eat like a slim person—you do. The point is that what you *believe* is reality.

That's a powerful tool; our reality manipulates our behavior. But hypnosis is not available to everyone. Nor should we routinely use it to change our behavior. It would, however, be truly wasteful to leave the power of belief untapped—there must be another way to harness it. Enter goals.

When you set goals and reach them, you use a process similar to hypnosis. On a conscious level, goals make you a believer by motivating you with explicit pictures of what you're working toward and by demonstrating your ability to reach them. All successful enterprises—corporations, governments, universities—use goals this way. Even more profound are goals' unconscious effects. Like hypnosis they work silently—you are completely unaware of what's happening while they steer your mind.

STIMULATING YOUR REWARD PATHWAY

Over the ages, the human brain evolved as the most advanced and complex organism on Earth. With it evolved a process that fosters the advancement of humankind by allowing us to reach beyond ourselves. Much of this process remains a mystery. But scientists have discovered the area of the brain involved with it: a distinct train of nerves running through its right and left hemispheres. To describe it, they named it the reward pathway.

Reward is a fitting name as this pathway is the mastermind behind all feelings of pleasure. Whenever you accomplish something, you feel satisfied. It's a pleasant feeling, and by no means a random occurrence because the reward pathway sponsored it. As a sponsor, your reward pathway thrives. Each time you attain a goal you stimulate your pathway to give you a pleasant feeling. But one goal is not enough. The reward pathway wants to be stimulated again and again, so it demands you to attain more goals. So strong is its demand, that it enlists the help of other areas of the brain—all outside of our conscious control. Knowledge and experience buried deep in our memories comes forth to aid our decision making. Suddenly an idea dawns, a problem is solved, and a goal is attained. Just as your body digests its food, the reward pathway digests each goal, working tirelessly to help you attain it. Your reward pathway, however, is no altruist. It oversees goal attainment, not to help you, but to ensure that it gets stimulated again. Altruist or not, this is a powerful partner.

Goal attainment is intrinsic stimulation: something you've done has naturally stimulated your pathway. Cocaine and heroin are unnatural stimulators. But unnatural does not mean ineffective. Users become slaves to the demands of their reward pathways, and they continue to stimulate it by taking drugs—even when they desperately want to stop. It's a sad scenario that teaches us a lesson: anyone can also extrinsically stimulate their reward pathway.

This obviously is not encouragement to take drugs; there are many other nonhabit-forming stimulators, namely, anything that gives you pleasure or enjoyment. These extrinsic stimulators, more commonly known as rewards, are powerful, but only if you earn them. By earning them you add value, and value is an essential ingredient; without it, a reward wouldn't stimulate your pathway. For years businesses have used rewards. Noticing a connection between rewards and performance, they give bonuses and promotions to encourage more good work.

That isn't to say you should wait for others to reward you. As long as you earn them, they should have as much—probably more—value as they would have if someone else gives them to you. This puts you in the driver's seat. I know an accounting supervisor who spent a lifetime working for a hard-nosed company that offered little advancement for the careers of its employees and even less appreciation for their work. It was a harsh stance, but the company got away with it. Situated in a rural area, it held many of its employees because of the limited local opportunities; if they wanted another job, they'd have to relocate. "I can't wait to retire and get out of this place," he'd often say. But he did wait and wait and wait to retire, counting every year as it dragged by. Don't play this waiting game. Set goals now. Then couple extrinsic rewards with the intrinsic rewards you receive upon goal attainment, and you keep your reward pathway busy and hungry for more—exactly the way you want it.

THE GOAL-REWARD CIRCLE

A hungry reward pathway works for you. After each goal is attained, it pushes you to form another one. I call it the goal-reward circle (see Figure 2.1). You set a goal, reach it, and reward yourself, following it immediately with another goal, another campaign, and another reward.

A reward pathway is not a rare gift; you along with everyone else are born with one, and whether it's used properly or not depends solely on you. Some people already know how to use their reward pathways. Others must learn. Knowing that you must set goals is a head start in the learning process, but there's more to it. Just as you must feed your body the right foods, you must feed your reward pathway the right goals.

| Figure 2.1 | ***THE GOAL-REWARD CIRCLE*** |

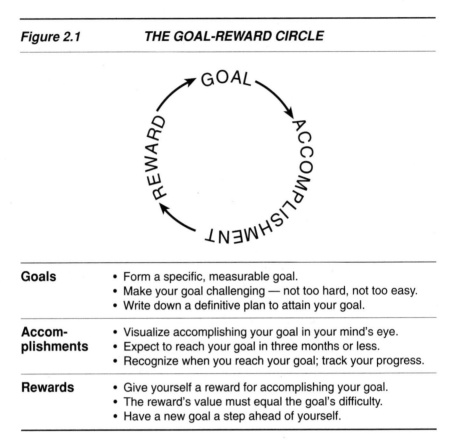

Goals	• Form a specific, measurable goal.
	• Make your goal challenging — not too hard, not too easy.
	• Write down a definitive plan to attain your goal.
Accom-plishments	• Visualize accomplishing your goal in your mind's eye.
	• Expect to reach your goal in three months or less.
	• Recognize when you reach your goal; track your progress.
Rewards	• Give yourself a reward for accomplishing your goal.
	• The reward's value must equal the goal's difficulty.
	• Have a new goal a step ahead of yourself.

Begin with a Clear Goal

To use all your knowledge, experience, and creativity for pursuing a goal, you must tell your brain *exactly what you want*. Be clear and specific. This not only creates a detailed picture of your goal; it allows you to vividly see yourself reaching it. Picturing your goal repeatedly shifts your reward pathway into high gear. But often people neglect clarity. They don't realize it's needed for a successful outcome, or they don't want to make the effort—it's easier to reach for a vague goal like happiness. This mistake mars many a personal and professional life. A consolidations manager, who was especially prone to panic, told his employees to revise two pages of an annual report without explaining exactly what he wanted done or delegating to each employee a specific task. The result: chaos with the wrong outcome. With such vague goal setting, a style that marked his management, he couldn't use his resources effectively. Eventually he was fired.

Even executives who use goals effectively at work stumble when transferring that skill to their personal lives. Faced with the challenge of becoming fit, they form a goal of simply becoming fit, with no dietary regimen, no exercise schedule, and no record keeping to tell them when they have reached turning points. Can you imagine running a business without record keeping? With goals like this, their reward pathways might as well retire.

But early retirement is not something your reward pathway wants. What it wants are the goals. Let's assume your goal is to become fit or to lead a heart-healthy life. Although the second goal is more specific than the first, it is still too vague to form a goal-reward circle. Both goals are impossible to picture. Yet despite this, they seem, at first, to work, solidifying your bad habit of aiming at vague goals that leave you confused over your eventual failure. These goals, however, were never effective. What propelled you forward in the beginning was the initial enthusiasm over your decision to become fit, not the goals. (See Figure 2.2 for examples of bad goals.)

Figure 2.2   *EXAMPLES OF BAD GOALS*

To join a gym and work out.	To pump some iron.
To exercise more often.	To get healthy, lean, and mean.
To make my diet healthier.	To relax a little more at work.
To lose some weight.	To be cool toward incompetence.
To drink less alcohol.	To not let the kids get to me.

Enthusiasm has a power of its own. Alone, it can perform seemingly monumental feats. Take the soldier who marches off to war. Initially, he is full of patriotism and enthusiasm—an ideal attitude for a member of a fighting force. But a stint in the trenches tests this enthusiasm, pitting it against the stress of battle, where it fades without the support of a clear cause (goal). To a soldier lacking enthusiasm, the fight seems pointless, and his morale plummets, decreasing his effectiveness. What does war have to do with getting fit? Every facet of getting fit involves changing habits, some of which have been with you since childhood and are not about to step aside. Talk about a battle. Yet with clear goals this battle is reduced to a mere skirmish easily won.

When your goal is clear and specific, your goal-reward circle takes over where your enthusiasm left off. A newcomer to exercise might set a specific goal to walk 20 minutes a day five days a week for three weeks in a row. Add the time of day and where you're going to walk, and you have full detail. A specific goal is trackable, meaning that progress toward it can be judged. Whenever you set a goal ask yourself, "Can I measure my progress toward it?" If the answer is no, the goal is not specific enough.

Can You Really Reach Your Goal?

Another requirement for goals is that they be reachable. If your goal is too far away, too difficult to attain, you will fail to reach it, breaking the goal-reward circle and seriously stunting your chances of reaching other goals. Pie-in-the-sky goals are as common as vague ones. How many people have starved themselves on too drastic a diet? How many people have plunged into too strenuous an exercise program? The answer is millions. Always set goals that are realistic and reachable; otherwise, you set yourself up for failure.

Also implicit here is that you be able to reach your goal in a reasonable amount of time. To be able to complete a marathon after running for one year might be reasonable, but one year is too long to wait. What do you get for your efforts while that year crawls by? Not enough according to your reward pathway. Meanwhile, on that far-off horizon, your goal dims. Set your goals so they can be reached within three months. This allows for unexpected delays and keeps your goal from obsolescing. (See Figure 2.3 for examples of good short-range goals.)

Not that goals should be a cinch to reach immediately either. While your goal must be reachable, it must also be demanding enough to qualify as a worthwhile accomplishment. Remember your reward pathway is watching—trying to slip an easy goal by won't work because it doesn't have enough value and value is what stimulates this pathway. You get what you work for.

Figure 2.3	**EXAMPLES OF GOOD SHORT-RANGE GOALS**

Cardio

Walk 1 mile in less than 22 minutes three times a week for three weeks in a row.

Jog 2 miles in less than 18 minutes three times a week for three weeks.

Cross-country ski at 5 kilometers per hour for 30 minutes three times a week for three weeks.

Give up smoking as of (date).

Muscular

Do a strength-building exercise for 20 minutes three times a week for six weeks.

Do as many push-ups as you can every other day for three weeks.

Do 40 continuous sit-ups six days a week for three weeks.

Do 10 minutes of stretching for hamstrings, back, chest, and neck three times a week for six weeks.

Nutrition

Substitute one low-fat item for one high-fat item in your diet each week (e.g., pretzels for potato chips).

Take a multivitamin, beta-carotene, vitamin E and vitamin C daily (women take folic acid daily; men take aspirin every other day).

Eat two servings of oat bran or oatmeal two times per week for one month then three times per week for one month and then five times per week for one month.

Stress

Practice abdominal breathing two times a day for 3 minutes at a time five days a week for four weeks.

Practice "staying in the present" for 3 minutes two times a day six days a week for three weeks.

Do a 5-minute muscular relaxation exercise as soon as you get to work each morning and immediately after lunch for three weeks.

For news "junkies," tune to the Weather Channel or sports news instead of the evening news six days a week for three weeks.

Attitude

Immediately upon waking up, visualize something positive transpiring over the course of the day seven days a week for three weeks.

Compliment the work or personal appearance of an employee once a day five days a week for four weeks.

Offer positive advice or help to one person each day without missing an opportunity for two weeks.

An Example of Setting Goals

It was the last Saturday of February, and all signs of winter were disappearing. As Ed, general counsel of his corporation, sat in his office working, he couldn't help noticing runners racing by his office building. He'd seen races before. But for Ed, that morning's observation was an awakening. He had wanted to start an exercise program all winter, and seeing those runners stirred his competitive spirit. Ed decided he was going to run races.

Running competitively is a sport that demands a certain level of fitness—before racing a 5-K or 10-K you need a minimum running base of two to three months. Knowing this, Ed asked a runner friend when some spring races would be held and found out there was a 10-K on May 2. That gave him nine weeks to prepare.

Ed bought a pair of running shoes and drew up a training program. For the first week's training, he would run 2 miles a day with a quarter-mile walk between them. The second week, he planned daily runs of 3 miles walking after the second mile, and the third week daily runs of 3 miles without stopping. The fourth week would be his biggest hurdle: 4 consecutive miles each day. Ed's goal each week was to complete his training as planned, but to complete seven 4-mile runs in a row was the goal that shined the brightest.

He accomplished his goal of running all seven days the first week. Then he ran on only five days of the next week; one day was lost because of snow, the other because of cold rain. His second week's goal was never really reached. But that didn't stop Ed from moving on to his third week's plan, and the next day he ran 3 consecutive miles—too much too soon. The impatience cost him. After that run, he was so sore that he not only rested the next day, but the next six days. Then he resumed his training with runs of one mile a day for a week. At that point Ed was doing a juggling act with his goals, pushing them back by revising his running distance downward. The only goal he didn't change was the one to run the race in May.

The rest allowed Ed to recover, and he started week 5 running 2 miles a day, increasing it to 3 miles toward the end of the week. Week 6's training consisted of 3-mile runs every other day. It was designed as an "off" week. This time Ed was listening to his mentor, who warned him not to push himself too hard. So he followed his plan and achieved his weekly goals—in fact he achieved two goals each week. One goal was to run pain free. The other was to follow his running schedule, and not push himself too far.

As Ed continued to run his enthusiasm grew, which encouraged him to reach for higher goals. These urges he managed to fight off until week 7. In the middle of that week, Ed ran an unplanned 6 miles just to show himself he could do it, and then rested the next three days. Impromptu as this goal was, it felt like—and really was—a milestone. Ed hadn't run six consecutive miles since high school. Now his goal to run the race was more important than ever.

Back to running in week 8, he logged in 4 miles each day. But the urge to test himself won again, and on the last day, he ran 5 miles instead of four. Again he felt exhilarated—it was another goal reached.

During his final week of training, Ed ran only 3 miles every other day—a week before the race was no time to take chances—and he didn't let his mounting enthusiasm overrule his running schedule.

On May 2 Ed ran the 10-K race in a respectable time of 43 minutes and change. Later that day, exhausted and sore but filled with pride, he boarded a plane to attend a tax seminar in Dallas. The race was over; it was time to rest. Yet Ed couldn't stop thinking about racing again. At the race he had been handed a flier announcing a mid-June race—a new goal. He drew up a training schedule on the back of his seminar program and began to picture the race—where he would start and finish it, what streets he would run on, how fast he would run each mile. The more he thought about it, the more excited he got, and he left during an afternoon break to comb a nearby shopping mall for the best running shoes. The ones he bought cost ninety-nine dollars, nearly twice as much as most running shoes sold at that time. But he figured he had earned them, and he needed them for the future.

Last year Ed found his first pair of running shoes in his basement. More than a decade had passed since he'd worn them. Now Ed regularly runs 50 miles a week and is a familiar face at local races where he routinely wins his age group—and passes out fliers for the next race.

Ed was lucky: he used goals even though he wasn't really aware that he was doing it. When he told me his story, he emphasized how carefully he planned his training schedule. Left in the background was the fact that he regularly set goals for himself to reach. Terms like milestone, successful week, confidence building, and turning point sprinkled his conversation, but the only time he ever used the word "goal" was as a reference to the race itself. Whether he knew it or not, his interim goals were propelling him forward. He also set an excellent main goal: only nine weeks away, specific and attainable (he had enough time to get into shape), known by his friends, easy to remember—the perfect vehicle to success.

Setting goals correctly requires knowledge and experience. Don't expect miracles from your first effort. Remember the goal-reward circle is repetitive, and its feedback will tell you whether your goals are too easy or too challenging. From it you'll learn to adjust your current goals and to set later ones more accurately—just like Ed.

Accomplishing Your Goal

After forming your goal, set out to accomplish it. This is a step-by-step process. With a specific goal, this process is easier to plan and monitor so you can recognize how far you've gone and when you've succeeded. But recognizing an accomplishment is not always easy, especially when it concerns ourselves. Distracted by activities that pull us in every direction, we often overlook gradual changes in our bodies or lifestyles.

Joan, a coworker, had been lifting weights for two months. "During that time," she said, "I figured my only gain was calluses on my hands. Then I went to the supermarket for a bag of charcoal. Well, I picked up a bag that looked to be the 20-pound size and put it in my cart, but it was so easy to carry that I checked the weight. Sure enough it was 20 pounds. That was the first evidence of my new strength." What about her workouts—hadn't she been making the weight progressively heavier? "Oh yes, but that was only during my workouts, and for some reason I never equated it with my body getting stronger." Is Joan an extreme example of inattentiveness? Unfortunately no. Part of the problem was her goal to "just get stronger." Too vague to give her any direction, it didn't tell her where she was going and therefore gave her no idea of what signs to look for on the way. A 20-pound bag of charcoal had to tell her. The other part of her problem is that she ignored evidence of her increasing strength during her workouts, as if it wasn't an accomplishment worthy of recognizing. Many people are brought up to believe that it's wrong to celebrate their accomplishments, so they pay heavy homage to modesty, downplaying their successes or even denying them. Notice your triumphs, large and small. If you can't tell whether you've reached your goal, stop, reset it, and start again.

Rewarding Your Accomplishment

Unconsciously, the reward pathway rewards you for attaining a goal by giving you a pleasant feeling of accomplishment. This is an intrinsic reward. Consciously, you can enhance an intrinsic reward by giving yourself something of value, an extrinsic reward. An extrinsic reward gives you the most control. You decide what it is and when you're getting it. But its timing is crucial; decide on an extrinsic reward when you set your goal. To put off choosing an extrinsic reward is to cheat yourself of the push it gives you toward your goal.

Always choose a specific reward. Don't say, "Well, I'll just relax." How are you going to relax? Where are you going to relax? A specific reward, like a specific goal, has more drawing power. It's easier to picture and therefore easier to imagine getting, which increases its power as an incentive.

But *you* must pick it out. Sometimes people work toward rewards from others. A raise, a promotion, a romance all fall under this rubric. Promises from others aren't fact—they may not come or they may not be what you expected. After working hard toward your goal, the last thing you need is a disappointment, which turns what should have been positive feedback into negative feedback. Extrinsic rewards may mean from the outside, but that "outside" must still be you.

Another requirement of an extrinsic reward is that it match the effort expended to reach the goal. A huge reward not earned gives as little pleasure as a small reward overexpended for. But it is not a black-and-white issue. How much you value rewards and the effort needed to earn them depends on your attitude and your knowledge. Does exercising 20 minutes a day, five days a week, for three weeks in a row represent a big accomplishment? Many new exercisers, impatiently eyeing the grand scheme of fitness, would say no. I say yes. Less than one-fourth of the population of the United

States exercises, despite the fact that a large portion knows it should—a statistic that adds value to any fitness accomplishment. Celebrate reaching small fitness goals with decent rewards. Fitness is that important.

Rewards come in many different forms. In my case, the ultimate reward is reading time, although food rewards are also high on my list. Not everyone would agree with me. What rules reward choosing is values, income, and location. If you enjoy music, for example, you might reward yourself by buying a set of CDs, or a CD player, or tickets to a concert. Or you could buy books, clothing, fishing gear, even weekends away. Jerry, an engineer and long-time runner, celebrates running 10 K's under 39 minutes with a splurge at the donut shop, temporarily ending his moratorium on eating those high-fat treats. For him there isn't a sweeter reward.

And don't overlook the greatest reward of all: doing something for someone else. A writer friend celebrated getting a book published by writing a check to her favorite charity. Another friend completed a marathon and gave his wife, who had cheered him on throughout his grueling training, a pair of gold earrings. Whenever you reach a fitness goal, try celebrating by getting someone else into exercise. There isn't a greater gift you can give. What you do depends on the needs of those around you and the rest of the world.

Still, no matter what the reward, the pleasure is only temporary. To be truly successful, you must keep moving forward, always looking for ways to improve yourself and the lives of those around you. Many people miss this point. They strive for a goal only to become disillusioned or depressed when they reach it. Where, they wonder, are all the fireworks of everlasting happiness? Their mistake was not in setting the goal, but in stopping when they reached it and expecting the fireworks to go on forever.

Such was the case with Angelo, a 42-year-old accountant. "I've worked so hard to build my own business," he said, "and now that I have a sizable clientele I'm still not happy. In fact, I'm not even sure I want to do this work anymore." Abandoning his business and starting over in another field was not an option. But setting new goals was. An avid weight lifter in college, Angelo joined a local gym to regain his old form: goal number one. As he got back into shape, however, he became interested in other exercises—running, rowing, stairclimbing. One goal led to another. Angelo began to read about nutrition. Today he still has his accounting business, but he is investigating ways to work nutrition into it. His latest goal: spread the word on fitness.

Your body and mind have almost limitless potential for growth and improvement—the reason why our reward pathway won't work if we stand still. Consider that a blessing and a warning. Don't rely on past successes to sustain your happiness. Let new goals show the way.

GOALS NEVER END

A circle has no beginning or end; its form makes it perpetual. The goal-reward circle revolves from a goal to an accomplishment to a reward and around again to another goal, another accomplishment, another reward. It too is perpetual. But where do all these revolutions go? Where do they take you? Goals are not mutually exclusive: every goal you achieve pushes you toward another goal, moving you closer to a long-range goal, be it a target weight or a marathon. Therefore the goal-reward circle is always revolving toward a higher goal. To picture this better, imagine reaching into the circle and pulling out a goal; along with it will come an accomplishment and reward, completing its own circle. Now reach in and pull out another goal and its partners. If you keep doing this, you'll soon have a stack of circles forming a spiral that begins with a commitment and ends with a long-range goal (see Figure 2.4). Movement up and around this spiral represents progress.

Moving toward a long-range goal is similar to taking a voyage. When you set sail, you know the course, which usually includes stops at several ports for interest and variety. But during the cruise you must sail according to the winds, adjusting as they shift in direction and velocity. The same is true of reaching a long-range goal. Stop off at short-range goals, while adjusting for unexpected events on the way.

Long-range goals don't have to be specific, but the short-range goals that form its spiral do. If, for example, you have a long-range cardio goal of running over 30 miles a week, approach it with short-range goals of shorter daily jogs that lengthen progressively, not with biking or rowing. Though these are good exercises and can be done while you train for running, they cannot become so prominent

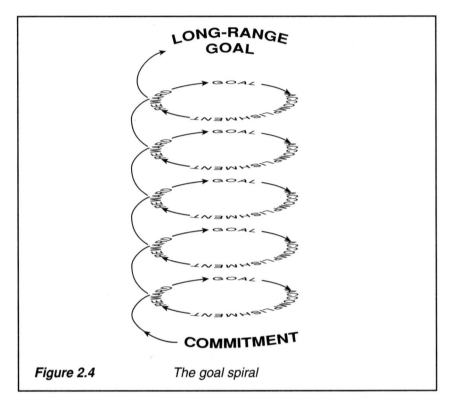

Figure 2.4   *The goal spiral*

in your program that they interfere with progress toward the long-range goal. If short-range goals clash, shift the one aimed at your long-range goal to a higher priority.

Expect a long-range goal to take between one and five years to reach. Because these goals usually relate to significant changes in lifestyle that require gradual uptake, enough time is needed to achieve them. In the area of fitness, rapid changes seldom hold. Attitude, nutrition, stress resilience are especially slippery; they change momentarily, giving you the impression that the battle is won. But this change is only a diversion. Lurking just beyond it are old attitudes, eating habits, and stress responses eagerly waiting to return if given an opportunity.

The other fitness components, cardio and muscular, are just as stubborn about sudden shifts from the status quo. Plunging into a strenuous exercise program almost guarantees you'll end up a refugee of exercise, sitting on the sidelines with nothing to show for the experience but a bad taste in your mouth and a bad opinion in your mind. You're not happy about it, but your old habits are. Never convinced that they'd completely lost their hold on you, these habits waited patiently until you were ripe for a relapse. Under the stress of an overly ambitious program, it doesn't take long to ripen. Then your sedentary habits comfortably reinstall themselves into your life. Some people, however, may be stubborn enough—or desperate enough—to withstand old habits, and they plug on with teeth-clenching persistence. For these "tough cases" old habits engage an ally: injury.

Long-range goals insert a patience factor that greatly increases your chances for success. Suppose you want to decrease your fat intake from 50 percent of your total calories to 25 percent. Do you plan to do it in a matter of weeks or months? I hope not. Any dietary change, from cutting fat and cholesterol to adding fluids and complex carbohydrates, takes a long time to install into your repertoire of habits. Bypass a long-range goal for this change and you'll doom yourself to failure.

Will you also fail at exercise if you don't have a long-range goal? That depends on what you want to do. The main purpose of a long-range goal is to give you direction and perspective. Whether you sail through a calm world or get blown off course by a gale wind, your long-range goal will be there as your guiding light. Illness, family problems, business crises—no one is immune to them. When beset by problems that shake up your short-range goals, look to your lighthouse. It will keep you on course (see Figure 2.5).

Short-range goal circles and long-range goal spirals are a simplified representation of how goals work. In real life, there are no endings, no final destinations. Each time you achieve a long-range goal, you replace it, spring-boarding from one spiral to another. But life is more complex than that. Often you'll be working in different stages of several spirals at the same time. This your brain can manage—and wants to. Multiple-goal spirals add balance, variety, and flexibility to your life. For example, if a heavy travel schedule interferes with your running goals, you can still work on your dietary goals. Therefore you still move toward your dietary goal, with the added bonus that you are also moving toward your running goal. A

Figure 2.5	*EXAMPLES OF GOOD LONG-RANGE GOALS*
Cardio	Maintain your heart rate at 60 percent of your VO_2 max for 1 hour comfortably.
	Lower your diastolic blood pressure by 10 milimeters of Hg.
Muscular	Double your strength and increase your flexibility so you can easily maintain stretching exercises for 30 seconds.
Nutrition	Regularly eat 60 percent of your daily calories from carbohydrates, 25 percent from fat, and 15 percent from protein (except for designated celebrations).
Stress	Feel less taxed and stressed out by occupational situations so you can enjoy your work more.
	Put family situations in their proper perspective and deal with them without anger.
Attitude	Possess a positive and optimistic attitude toward your present accomplishments and future possibilities.

---

low-fat, high-carbohydrate diet reinforces an endurance exercise like running. Not all long-range goals fit together as well as these two, but having multiple-goal spirals does give you options when conflicts arise.

Making the Pledge

Once you decide on your goals, you have to manage them. Here long-range goals present a special challenge: their long distance from you threatens them with obsolescence. You might even forget them. Your goals are the future you want. Keep them alive by using a time-proven method of organizing multiple and complex tasks: write them down. Record long- and short-range goals in a planning diary or logbook and refer to it often. Thinking about (but not worrying about) your goals, you push yourself consciously and unconsciously toward them. A forgotten goal is no goal at all.

Another way of securing your goals is to tell someone else about them. Choose someone who is also interested in fitness: a friend, the fitness pro at your corporate gym, even a member of a running club. Running clubs are the most common athletic club. They are located in many cities and towns across the United States, and are open to all exercisers, not just runners. As a nonrunning member, just being around other exercisers will benefit you. And runners, in particular, are very supportive of many different fitness goals.

If there aren't any running clubs nearby or any exercise minded friends around, tell anyone who will listen: your spouse, your boss, your doctor, your hair stylist. But whoever you tell, first make sure that the person is sympathetic. Nothing puts a damper on a goal like a pessimistic person: "You'll get hurt." "Where will you get the time for that?" "I know someone who smoked, drank, never exercised, and still lived to 100." Such comments are worse than no response. Anyone can be a confidant, but you must still choose him or her carefully.

An excellent confidant is a personal trainer. Knowledgeable about many facets of exercise, he can steer you by the pitfalls and point you toward the future. A personal trainer is a gold mine of exercise knowledge from whom you can dig out experience that would take you years to accumulate. Obviously, the services of a personal trainer are not free, but they are well worth the investment. Still, no one should need a personal trainer for longer than two months. There is just so much you can learn from one person. At some point your own curiosity will kick in and lead you to articles and books on subjects relevant to your physical talents and exercise goals.

DOING IT FOR YOURSELF

Aim a series of short-range goals at a distant objective and you have a goal spiral. Goal spirals are the core of your fitness campaign. Some components of fitness might have one spiral; others might have several. Together they form a network of spirals, different for each person because no two people have the same strengths and weaknesses. But all people bind their spiral network with the same kind of mattress—their attitude.

Attitude colors your world, and it can be the difference between the success or failure of your fitness program. Do you truly value a heart-healthy lifestyle, or are you under doctor's orders? Do you believe that fitness leads to success by improving you or by impressing others? Do you want to live the longest, most active life possible, or just the longest one possible? With the wrong attitude, your program doesn't stand a chance.

What affects your attitude most is the one you are doing all this for. If you see fitness as a way to please a spouse or loved one, if you want to show a friend what you are made of, if you think you can dress up your work record to impress your boss, you are doing it for the wrong person. A self-improvement program, especially a long-term one, must be done for yourself. Alcoholics Anonymous, Narcotics Anonymous, and Overeaters Anonymous are groups that have proven this many times; members who join them to please someone else usually fail. Like these programs, getting fit requires a sizable change in behavior. On the surface it might seem that pleasing someone else, a very important someone else, is the same as pleasing yourself. But to your brain it isn't. Again, you cannot fool your reward pathway. A response from someone else seldom matches what you expected, and its power to stimulate your reward pathway is muted by this disparity. Granted, the other person may wholeheartedly want you to make the positive changes in your lifestyle, but you are not the center of their universe. They are. Your accomplishments they can appreciate only to a certain degree, and they will express that appreciation to a lesser degree than that. Even the most enthusiastic supporters won't praise you forever. They can't; they have their own lives to lead, just as you have your life to lead, your universe to be the center of.

No one else can give you the same feeling you get when you reach a goal for yourself. Nor can they applaud you at the right time. When you achieve a goal for yourself, there is no waiting for the adulation of others; your reward pathway knows immediately.

Your fitness goals are too important to rely on the opinion of others. "All day long I answer to others—my boss, my wife, my kids," a friend said recently. "Working out I feel alive and free. It's the one thing I do totally for myself." Ask yourself what *you* want to do. Then do it.

• CHAPTER 3 •

CREATING TIME FOR FITNESS

At medical school orientation we were told that after one week we'd be a month behind and never catch up. It was true. The course load was equivalent to 30 graduate credits each semester, a schedule almost impossible to manage sanely. Some students got depressed; others just got drunk. But not Paul—he remained positive and focused. How did he withstand the intense pressure of medical school? He ran: almost every day, up and down Manhattan's First Avenue and through its East Side neighborhoods. This mystified me. Where did he find the time to run when I hardly had enough time to eat and sleep? "I find a little time here and there," he would say, "and besides, after I run I feel recharged. I can study better and get more done." Paul graduated from medical school number one in the class.

As an executive, you manage impossibly tight schedules too. But evidence suggests you don't "find a little time here and there" for personal fitness. And if you don't have the time, you don't have a chance.

Faced with this dilemma you may wonder: exactly how did Paul do it? It's a valid question. This chapter will answer the question by showing you how to create time in three ways: first, by changing your sleep habits; second, by being more efficient, doing the same activities in less time; and third, by EXTRAcising, getting "extra" tasks done while you exercise.

Creating time is one of the most rewarding problems you'll ever solve. It will free you to change your life. But, first check your attitude. Are you committed to total fitness? Even if you already exercise a little, are you ready to take that commitment to a higher level? The answers must be yes.

Once you identify with fitness it will be easier to find the time for it. Can you imagine if Larry Bird never found time to practice free throws? To him fitness was more than a job or sport, it was his identity, so he made it a priority. And so should you make fitness a priority because it affects you in every way, including how successful you are in your career and family life. Fitness isn't an addition to your life; it *is* your life.

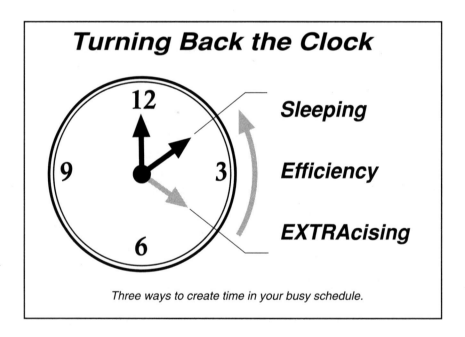

Turning Back the Clock

Sleeping

Efficiency

EXTRAcising

Three ways to create time in your busy schedule.

HOW YOUR SLEEPING HABITS TAKE TIME

With the right attitude in place, you can do anything. Now you are ready to create fitness time. Consider a typical day in your life. What is the largest block of time you have control over? It is while you sleep..

Although research has shown that the amount of sleep needed varies from person to person, it has also shown that most people need less sleep than they get. In fact, too much sleep sets you up for problems. It makes it harder to fall asleep and stay asleep, a predicament that makes you think you need more sleep, instead of less. What seems like a healthy rest is really a bad habit.

How Much Sleep Do You Need?

Examine your sleeping habits. Do you get over seven hours of sleep a night? If you do, you are probably getting too much. But don't respond by setting your alarm an hour earlier or going to bed an hour later. You are changing a habit, and it should be done gradually. Start by waking up 15 minutes early. Do not shorten your sleeping time by going to bed later; that will only gain you less productive evening hours when your system is literally winding down. Always aim for the morning hours.

After two weeks of waking up 15 minutes early, set your alarm 15 minutes earlier. Now you've gained a half hour. Does your body miss the sleep? No. The body, excluding the brain, doesn't need sleep, and the brain, which does need sleep, has, over a few weeks, gradually grown used to getting less of it. But don't stop here. You are experimenting to find out how much sleep you really need, so carve out another 15 minutes by getting up earlier. Just remember to give yourself two weeks to get used to each cutback in sleep. By the time you're waking up an hour early, you'll be wondering why you ever wanted to sleep that late because what you are doing with that extra hour is far more refreshing.

Implicit here is the point that your sleep habits must be consistent—that you go to bed the same time each night and wake up the same time each morning. Weekend departures from your regular weekday sleeping patterns are, within limits, acceptable. But crashing at 3:00 A.M. and waking up at 11:00 A.M. is unhealthy. It disrupts your circadian rhythms. Such disruptions—especially those related to sleep—can cause depression. By wrenching your sleep cycle and circadian rhythms violently with weekend activities, you invite a minidepression that strikes on Monday morning and may last well into Tuesday. Unfortunately, people with these Monday blues blame the day—"It's Monday"—instead of themselves.

The cure is simple: on weekends, do not sleep more than a half hour longer than you do on weekdays. This rule, however, does not apply during extremely stressful times at work. Your brain needs the extra rest, so by all means get it on weekends. Just don't make it a habit. If it already is a habit, break it—fast. Throughout this book I endorse changing habits slowly. But here you are correcting a problem for your body; the faster you do it, the better. (See Figure 3.1 for a review of changing your sleep habits.)

Figure 3.1	**CHANGING YOUR SLEEP HABITS**
Weekdays	Wake up 15 minutes earlier for a two-week period. Wake up another 15 minutes early for another two weeks. Continue this progression until you wake up 1 hour earlier.
Weekends	Crashing late at night and waking up late disrupts your circadian rhythms. Keep your weekend sleep pattern within a half hour of your weekday pattern. It will promote quality sleep and eradicate Monday morning blues.

Sleeping Peacefully

Ultimately this may mean changing some social habits. But you will gain more than time by doing it. When you change sleep habits to appease your circadian rhythms, you improve your performance while awake and the quality of your rest while asleep. Higher quality sleep means falling asleep faster and sleeping more soundly. Six hours of sound sleep, for example, is as refreshing as seven or eight hours of fragmented sleep; it leaves you feeling as though you slept that extra hour.

Still, cutting back on sleep won't affect everyone in the same way. If you regularly feel sleepy during the evening, go to bed 15 minutes early. That preserves your newfound time in the morning. As far as the time you lose in the evening, that tends to be filled with snacking and watching the nightly news. You don't need the calories or the tragedies. Avoiding exposure to upsetting or angering information before bed will improve the quality of your sleep.

But you can be your own worst enemy by trying to improve sleep quality through self-treatment with alcohol and over-the-counter medications. One of the most common "cures" for sleeping problems is alcohol, which superficially appears to work. Many people feel more relaxed and even sleepy under the influence of modest to moderate amounts of alcohol. In fact alcohol can help you fall asleep. Beyond that, the wolf takes off his sheepskin; even small amounts of alcohol will distort a person's sleep pattern. While you "sleep," the level of alcohol in your blood decreases and so does its sedating effects. Do you wake up right away? No, but you might as well; the lower level of alcohol in your blood can still fragment your sleep cycle. Typically you awaken many times during the night and spend little time in the deep-sleep cycle you need to function well throughout the day.

Trying over-the-counter preparations to remedy sleep problems is also futile. Most of these are benadryl or some other antihistamine medication, and they have the same effect on your sleep as alcohol. All distort your sleep cycle, quickly become ineffective, and cause a rebound insomnia that is usually worse than what you started with.

Another "over-the-counter" substance that affects the quality of your sleep is caffeine. Everyone knows caffeine can keep you awake, but what most people don't know is that it lasts a lot longer than they think. While it will keep you awake for only one to one and a half hours, it will stay in your system and disrupt your sleep for up to five hours (see Figure 3.2). This may seem to be a paradox: something that can't keep you awake can disrupt your sleep anyway. But it's a matter of degree. The difference between the states of wakefulness and sleep is a big one; therefore it takes a comparatively big dose of caffeine to keep you awake. The difference between good and poor quality sleep is much more subtle. Your sleep architecture, the cycles of sleep you experience through the night, is a fragile thing. Even low levels of caffeine, not potent enough to keep you awake, can tear it apart.

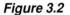
Figure 3.2   **CAFFEINE DISRUPTS SLEEP**

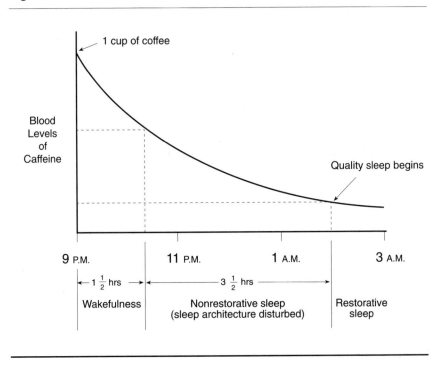

The most well-known caffeine carrier is coffee (80–150 mg per cup) and not far behind is tea (50–70 mg per cup) and many kinds of soft drinks, especially the colas (40–55 mg per 12-ounce can). If you're not sure whether something contains caffeine, check the ingredients. That includes the ingredients of medications. Certain brands of aspirin and other over-the-counter analgesics contain caffeine in significant amounts (50–100 mg per two-pill dose)—the pill you take for your aching back or headache can ruin half a night's sleep.

Daylight can also affect how much sleep you need. Can you recall those times in winter when you lack energy and motivation, crave sweets, and long for more sleep? You may have attributed these feelings to the "post holiday blues." In reality, they are a common response to the dwindling hours of daylight and the fading intensity of the sun during winters in latitudes north of North

Carolina. Occasionally people become severely depressed. But most of us simply eat and sleep more than usual. My prescription to ease this desire for more sweets and sleep is to get more sun: go out at midday without sunglasses for 30 minutes three or four times a week. At that time of day the sun's rays are most intense and they will inject some summer energy into your routine—including the need for less sleep.

Another way to adjust to less sleep is to take a nap. A 10- to 15-minute nap in the early afternoon recharges your brain, not by making up for lost sleep, but by giving it a rest when it needs it most. Between 2:00 P.M. and 3:00 P.M., the bodily rhythms slow down. A short nap then will renew your energy and creativity for the rest of your busy day. The business world may not be tuned into naps just yet, but in the near future, don't be surprised to find that more and more resourceful executives are using this technique to improve their stamina and increase their productivity.

Most people want to sleep more only because they think they need to. If you get quality sleep, you don't. Follow these guidelines and improve the quality of your sleep. Then sleep less, feel better, and enjoy the most peaceful time of day, morning.

WAYS TO FIND HIDDEN TIME IN EVERYDAY ACTIVITIES

To create even more time, be more efficient while you are awake: do your normal tasks in less time through planning and organizing. Planning and organizing—basic tenants in the business world. No doubt you are already familiar with these principles. But do you apply them consistently throughout your life? Though highly organized with your work time, you probably take a more lax approach to your personal time. Yet what you do with your time after work can dramatically affect what you accomplish with your time at work.

Examine your schedule. Even if you consider yourself organized, there are probably places in it that can yield more time. This, however, is not advice to organize every nanosecond of your life. Organizing smooths out your life. But taken too far it begins to have a life of its own, pushing you to organize, reorganize, and reorganize some more, and in the process you waste more time than you actually save—a perfect example of the law of diminishing returns.

The opposite attitude—that efficiency cannot possibly solve your time problem—is just as bad. Applying efficiency, even the busiest person can find time if he or she knows where to look.

Taking Time to Eat

Start with meals. Breakfast is all too often coffee and a roll or donut on your way to work. Can you possibly slice a wedge of time out of this meal? No, and you shouldn't try to. But you should at least make it healthy. An unhealthy breakfast can leave you dragging, and you can't be efficient if you're dragging—at home, at work, or anywhere else.

At lunch eat a light meal or snack. As long as it's nutritious, it's enough. A large meal eaten in a restaurant or cafeteria not only takes more time, but slows you down later in the day. If you are a big-lunch executive, gradually scale back over several weeks to a light lunch that takes only 15 minutes. Obviously, working lunches are exceptions, but you can still avoid alcohol, order light fare such as a salad, and do good business.

That brings us to dinner, the meal Americans spend the most time on. Dinner is a tradition worth preserving for its positive psychological impact—so keep the dinner hour sacred. But handle it efficiently. For many people, dinner devours too much time.

The first remedy is to move dinner back a half hour or more. If, for example, you eat at 6:00 P.M., delay dinner until 6:30 or 7:00 P.M. Family members who get home early, say, before 6:00 P.M., can fend off hunger with a light but nutritious snack. Again, a large meal slows you down, both in the time it takes to eat it and the effect it has on your mind and body. Usually it instigates a decline in your productivity, and you waste time after it.

Where you eat can also waste time. Eating out invariably uses more time than cooking the meal at home. First, it takes time to drive back and forth to a restaurant. Then you wait to eat and pay. And forget about fast-food restaurants saving you time; unless you hit them during a slack time, you'll end up waiting there too. As for cooking at home, a little planning saves you a lot of time. Cook meals in bulk and freeze them for individual dinners in the future. In the long run it saves time in set-up and clean-up of cooking, and defrosting a meal is as convenient as it gets. If you don't or won't cook, rely on the frozen food aisles of your supermarket. Just choose wisely.

What to Wear

With meals streamlined, your quest for efficiency should spur you to examine other everyday activities, where, hidden in cracks and crevices, are smaller pieces of time to be saved. Start with your morning routine. What are you going to wear to work? Or if you exercise first, what are you going to work out in? Both decisions are made more efficiently the night before because you tend to make decisions faster in the evening than first thing in the morning. And five minutes in the morning is more valuable than five minutes in the evening.

To make clothing decisions easier, organize your clothing by function: store work clothing separately from casual clothing and exercise clothing. True, it takes time and effort to initially organize your wardrobe, but in the long run it will save you far more time. Putting out clothing the night before will become a minute job, and gathering clothing for business trips will become a swift process that minimizes the chance of forgetting an important item.

Organize Your Shopping

Now that you've gotten your clothing in order, move on to another area where you can save time—shopping. Many people consider shopping a single activity, but included in it are many subactivities: driving, searching, appraising, waiting, paying, all rife with wasted time. How do you save time shopping? You drive less, search less, appraise less, and wait less; in short you organize yourself. Organized shoppers avoid shopping during peak hours, which cuts down on the waiting. They also know everything they need to buy before they leave the house, not because their memories are better, but because they make a list. Therefore, create a list center in a high-use room, such as the kitchen, where you can note items you need to buy. Include lists for all stores you shop regularly: the grocery store, pharmacy, bakery, hardware store, sporting-goods store. When your list is long, as it is for your weekly visit to the supermarket, write the items on your list in the same order as you walk through the store. This prevents you from missing items on your list and saves you the time of rereading it repeatedly. List-making drastically cuts down on extra shopping trips. It also enables you to link errands, which cuts down on your driving time.

Carpool for Children's Activities

Driving is something most executives spend too much time doing. If you have children, your driving obligations have probably reached crisis proportions. Recently a neighbor remarked, "My schedule revolves around my children's social lives." She is the rule, not the exception. Today, parents moonlight as chauffeurs for their children. Of course, some chauffeuring is necessary. But when it begins to drain your time and energy, take steps to change the situation. Form a car pool with parents whose children are involved in similar activities. Children seek activities that parents with much in common support; hence, it may be easier to form kiddy car pools than work car pools. By freeing yourself of half your chauffeuring duties, without sacrificing the peace of mind that your children are being safely transported, you can save much time. In fact, now you can finish activities that were once broken up by chauffeuring—no stopping and starting again. Another efficiency booster.

Watch Your Television Time

Time efficiency means getting a good return on your time investment. Nowhere do you get a worse return on your investment than when you watch TV. Both time efficiency experts and personal development authorities suggest that you minimize TV watching, worthy advice when you consider the fear and violence it injects into your life. Even the news is depressing. As parents, you are aware of the negative impact TV can have on your children. But have you noticed how it affects you? TV not only consumes your valuable time; it frequently leaves you in a downbeat emotional state. In that condition you cannot function efficiently. Nor can you sleep restfully. Delete this programming from your schedule; it will keep your spirits higher and free up more time in the evening.

There is, however, another side to TV; it can provide funny and intellectually stimulating programs. Sporting events, too, have an inspirational effect on people. Still, it takes time to watch these programs. Save some of that time by taping on your VCR. With the program taped you can watch it at your convenience—not during your prime time—and fast forward through commercials. TV programs sometimes offer good entertainment. Commercials never do. (See Figure 3.3 for a summary of efficiency ideas.)

Figure 3.3	**EFFICIENCY: FINDING HIDDEN TIME**
Breakfast	Spend a few extra minutes. Eat more. Eat nutritiously. This improves performance.
Lunch	Stop eating large meals; snack instead. Over a period of weeks gradually cut back to a 15-minute lunch.
Dinner	Move dinner back 30 to 60 minutes. Eat at home. Cook meals in bulk and freeze in individual servings.
Clothing	Decide what to wear the night before. Organize clothing by function: work, casual, exercise.
Shopping	Create a list center in a convenient location. Keep "living" lists. Use meaningful sequences with errands linked together.
Children	Share chauffeuring with parents of children's friends.
Television	Watch only cheerful, innovative, educational, sports programming. Use your VCR. Fast forward through commercials, clutter.

EXTRAcising Solves Exercising Conflicts

By using only a few tips in this chapter, you can create enough time to exercise. Still, some people may find it difficult to let go of other activities. EXTRAcising is the solution to this problem. EXTRAcising means doing something else while you exercise. Let's say, for example, that you cycle or cross-country ski indoors. Add reading racks—available with both kinds of equipment—and you can read and write. Carefully place tables, bookshelves, and entertainment centers around your exercise equipment, and you can reach a TV, a telephone, a VCR, a stereo system, tapes, books, journals, and writing materials without interrupting your exercise. Some exercises like rowing, running, and stairclimbing do limit your extra activities. But you can still watch TV or listen to your favorite music or continuing education or self-help tapes. Before you know it your workout will be over.

Above all, you can plan and solve problems while you do any exercise. Aerobic exercise especially helps you relax while it stimulates your creativity, two conditions that inspire your most inventive thinking. Many creative ideas originate during exercise sessions. What you accomplish with your mind is limited only by your goals.

All EXTRAcising is ultimately doing two activities at once. Exercise is always one of those activities. The other activity is anything your needs dictate. In effect you create time to exercise by exercising while you do one of your routine activities. (See Figure 3.4 for EXTRAcising examples.)

Figure 3.4   *EXTRACISING: ACTIVITIES WHILE YOU EXERCISE*

TV Viewing	Have a TV and VCR handy. Use remote controls.
Listening	Listen to your favorite music, continuing education, self-help tapes. Headphones are optional.
Reading	Pursue novels, mail, educational, cooking/recipes, vacation, and travel ideas.
Writing	Make lists of things to do and write down ideas for future projects.
Phoning	Return calls, set up appointments, shop, sell.
Conversing	Talk with spouse, children. Review the day's events. Discuss plans for holidays, meals, vacations, outings.

EXTRAcising Creates Family Time

EXTRAcising also covers family activities, and its healthful benefits for you and your children make it one of the best ways to spend time with them. In 1987 a government-sponsored panel estimated that less than 50 percent of all children exercised daily. Children are not immune to the ill effects of sedentary living. Exercise with them, and while you do that, find out what's going on at school, plan family outings and vacations—show them that they matter.

Anaerobic exercise especially lends itself to EXTRAcising because it's discontinuous bursts of activity broken up by periodic rests. Weight lifting, for example, is a popular anaerobic exercise that you can take turns doing with your children, who will love participating in an adult activity. No time is better spent. The exercise habit is one of the greatest gifts you can give your children.

HOW TO BEST USE THE EXTRA TIME YOU CREATE

As you sift through the strategies of EXTRAcising, gaining efficiency, and changing sleep habits, remember your objective of creating blocks of time for fitness. That some of the ideas in this chapter won't be feasible for you only confirms that no two lifestyles are alike. Your job is to use the ideas you can to chisel time out of your day for a fitness program. Obviously, not all of the time you create will be directly usable for fitness. The best time for that is before a meal, either in the morning, at noon, or in the evening. Therefore, you may need to rearrange some of your daily activities and then tailor your fitness program to fit the blocks of time you created.

A block of morning time between 30 and 60 minutes long is best used for aerobic exercise. Mornings tend to be quieter. Working out at this time, you are less likely to be disturbed or interrupted and more likely to feel relaxed and happy during a greater part of the day. It also helps you sleep better. In fact, morning exercise is used as therapy for depression and chronic insomnia.

What, then, should you do with newfound time if you already exercise in the morning? The answer is exercise more. Moderately active people are fitter than sedentary people; very active people are fitter than moderately active people. The fitter you are, the better. It's the best way to get an edge in today's highly competitive and stressful corporate environment.

Some pieces of time, however, are trickier to use than others. Time from your lunch hour is one of these. Unlike morning time, it is neither quiet nor guaranteed—meetings run into it, phone calls interrupt it, pressing projects upstage it. Still, some people will insist that it's the most convenient time to exercise. So they contort their schedules—and ultimately themselves—to squeeze in a walk, or run, or a trip to the gym. This makes exercise a stressor. Midday is *not* a good time to exercise if it means rushing or frequently skipping part or all of the workout. Exercise is a priority that you should enjoy, not a chore that you rush through.

Instead use "lunch" time for stretching and managing stress. It takes 40 seconds to stretch one muscle group and 5 minutes to stretch all large muscle groups below the waist, a workout that will prevent injuries, improve flexibility, ward off arthritic conditions, and relax your muscles—effects that spread to your mind. Now that's efficiency.

To relax your mind even more, practice stress management. Like stretching, managing stress fits into small pieces of time, and its payoff is tremendous. When done consistently, stress management techniques have a powerful, cumulative effect. The only time they don't work is when you don't do them.

Stretching and stress management are not mere underlings to formal exercise. They are integral parts of any fitness program and can be done on your lunch hour or at any other time of day.

That brings us to evening. Though not so private as morning time, 20 minutes or more before dinner is a good time to exercise aerobically. But an aerobic workout must be continuous—that is without interruptions. If you have children, fit into this time an anaerobic exercise, like weight lifting. Weight lifting lends itself to interruptions, which, depending on their ages, children can generously provide.

As for after-dinner time, avoid vigorous exercise. It stimulates you, and if done too close to bedtime, will keep you awake. Save this time for managing stress and stretching. These techniques soothe—exactly what you need before bedtime.

A fitness program is a lifestyle that places exercise, and taking care of yourself in general, on a pedestal high above life's other demands. People make time for it because they are hungry for better lives. So examine your habits, rearrange your activities, identify your problems, and watch for opportunities. Elevate yourself to a new level of organization and "find a little time here and there." Feed your body, your mind, and your career.

• CHAPTER 4 •

CHOOSING YOUR EXERCISE

My first 10-kilometer race was an exhilarating experience. It spiked my competitive juices; I had to race more and run faster. So I asked Sheila, a social worker friend and longtime racer, for advice. She suggested interval training: alternating sprints with jogs during the same workout. She also suggested I accompany her the next time she ran intervals, warning me that they were no fun to do alone.

Two days later we met at a high school track near the hospital where we worked. After warming up with a 2-mile jog, then carefully stretching our quads, hamstrings, and Achilles tendons, we tore off on our first interval. At first I glided along, striding forward with no effort at all. My breathing hit an easy rhythm that seemed to match that set by my arms and legs. But less than halfway through the sprint my running form collapsed. My breathing got louder and lapsed into irregular gasps for air. A burning sensation invaded my quads as my legs became almost too heavy to control. A tension spread down from my shoulders through my arms and hands. Even they began to tire. Finally I staggered over the finish line. But instead of jogging, I stopped, bent forward, leaned my hands on my knees, and gulped air. Still burning, my legs began to tremble. What happened?

Differences Between Aerobic and Anaerobic Exercise

My normally aerobic exercise, running, became anaerobic, and the difference was a big one. Yet I had actually done the exercise—though perhaps a bit too zealously—that would train me to run faster, and in doing so I had upheld a basic tenet of fitness: match the exercise to the goal. What are your goals? Do you want to improve your cardiovascular system? Do you want stronger muscles and bones? Or do you need work in all areas? Exercise, in general, is a vehicle to these goals, but no one exercise—that is, specific activity—can get you to them all.

To understand why, you have to know the difference between aerobic and anaerobic exercise. People unfamiliar with exercise physiology might think of aerobic exercise as a Jane Fonda aerobics class, bouncing through a percussion-driven workout. Well it is, but it's also much more. Aerobic exercise is any continuous, rhythmic movement of large muscle groups that can be maintained for more than a few minutes. Notice the words "continuous" and "maintained." They imply that you can keep exercising; that you're not within minutes or even seconds of working your muscles to their limit, that it is a low-intensity exercise. An exercise, therefore, is aerobic if its intensity is low enough to allow the muscles to use oxygen to produce the energy they need.

Raise the intensity enough, however, and the muscles must resort to producing energy without oxygen. This is anaerobic exercise. How, then, do you know when you have intensified your workout enough to cross the threshold from aerobic to anaerobic? Your muscles will tell you. They begin to burn, indicating the presence of lactic acid, a by-product of anaerobic energy production. Hence, whether an exercise is aerobic or anaerobic depends on the intensity with which you do it. A jog is aerobic. A trained runner can literally do it for hours. A sprint, as I found out with Sheila, is anaerobic. Once you feel the burn of lactic acid, you know your muscles can't go on at that intensity much longer.

Aerobic exercise is known as a heart-healthy activity. By enlisting large muscle groups, it disperses the work load, internally lowering the workout intensity. But these exercising muscles still burn more energy, which increases their need for oxygen. So they call the heart. Hearing this call, the heart starts pumping oxygen-rich blood faster. It becomes a cycle: the muscles keep working and demanding more oxygen; the heart keeps pumping hard and sending more blood. When the muscles exercise aerobically, the heart exercises too.

But a 5- or 10-minute workout won't do. To condition your heart, you must exercise for 20 minutes or more. A conditioned heart is a stronger heart; it can pump faster and push larger volumes of blood with each beat. It's also a heart with more blood vessels. Efficiency is a law in the human body, and if the heart is going to exercise regularly, it too will need a way to get more oxygen to feed its greater energy needs. From these new pipelines the heart can get it.

Besides developing the heart and circulatory capacity, aerobic exercise trains the skeletal muscles for greater energy production. Together these physical changes yield endurance, a quality that enables a cyclist to peddle dozens of miles or a runner to stride thousands of times. But it won't make the cyclist or runner strong. That is the job of anaerobic exercise.

Again, anaerobic exercise is intense. To forge enough intensity to build muscle size and strength, you must focus your effort on one small, distinct muscle group at a time. Weight lifting is a well-known anaerobic exercise. If the weights you lift are so light you can continue to lift them for over 12 repetitions, you don't work hard enough to quickly push your muscles into anaerobic energy production, and instead of building strength, you build endurance. As for the sprinters who accelerate that well-known aerobic exercise of running into the anaerobic realm, their thighs, particularly their quadriceps in the front, show the kind of exercise they've been doing. These are strong muscles built for short bursts of intense running. And they look it.

One muscle that doesn't get strong from anaerobic exercise is the heart. For the heart to benefit, it must work continuously for at least 20 minutes. But anaerobic exercise is too intense for such continuity; it requires repeated starts and stops, which literally interrupts your heart's workout. In fact, throughout an anaerobic workout, the heart is caught in a "Catch 22." Some lactic acid produced by the muscles leaks into the bloodstream and travels to the brain. Recognizing this by-product, the brain assumes more oxygen is needed. "Send more shipments of oxygen," it tells the heart, and the heart complies by beating faster. But more oxygen in the bloodstream is not the answer. The muscle that is releasing the lactic acid is working so hard, contracting so fiercely, it squeezes shut the very blood vessels that can deliver oxygen to it. With this downstream resistance to extra blood shipments, the blood pressure rises. Could this be dangerous? Not in a healthy person. If you want to exercise your heart, along with the rest of your cardiovascular system, exercise aerobically. If you want to build muscle and bone strength, exercise anaerobically. Both ways are safe.

Most exercises are classified as aerobic or anaerobic (see Figure 4.1) based on the muscles exercised and the normal intensity at which they are done. Following Figure 4.1 is an explanation of each exercise describing the muscles it uses and the pros and cons of doing it. This is to help you choose one that matches your goal. But don't choose by aerobic or anaerobic alone. Read each description carefully. Then imagine yourself doing it, filling in all the details you can: when, where, with whom. Does this scene feel comfortable to you? Do you think you can make it a habit? The more objective your answers, the better your chances of sticking with the exercise.

Figure 4.1   **AEROBIC AND ANAEROBIC EXERCISES**

Aerobic	Anaerobic (Weight Lifting)	
Walking	ABDOMINALS	SHOULDERS
Racewalking	Sit-ups	Side lifts
Running	Reverse trunk twists	Front lifts
Cross-country	BACK	LEGS
skiing	Reverse flies	Reverse leg lifts
Cycling	One-arm rowing	Weighted leg extensions
Aerobics	Back raises	Heel raises
Stairclimbing	CHEST	ARMS
Rowing	Supine flies	Dumbbell curls
Swimming	Barbell bench press	Tricep barbell curls
Circuit training		Kickbacks
		Push-ups

AEROBIC EXERCISES FOR YOU TO CONSIDER

WALKING/RACEWALKING. Walking is a good beginning exercise for people who have been inactive for a long time. As a gentle introduction to exercise, it is effective in forming an exercise habit—no refugee of exercise has ever claimed they overdid walking.

Working all the large muscles below the waist, walking, even at a moderate pace, tunes up your cardiovascular system. Turn up the speed and you sharpen the tune-up. A brisk walk easily becomes a very brisk walk and then a racewalk, elevating your heart rate to a better workout.

Of all the walking exercises, racewalking gives you the best workout. Though not as popular as running, it is a superb aerobic exercise almost as intense as running, and its nonjarring movement subjects the walker to little pounding, greatly reducing the chance of injuries.

But it's not just walking as fast as you can; racewalking has a specific technique. To learn it, simply buy an instruction video. Racewalking gives the same benefits as running, and it's an excellent choice for anyone with foot, knee or back problems.

RUNNING. Even more convenient than walking is running. With running, you can achieve the same cardio fitness in less time. That and its transportability—you can do it at home, at work, in another city—make it the most popular aerobic exercise. Running clubs, clinics, and races all give you regular contact with other runners. For those who don't need the socializing—you'd rather escape from the daily crush of humanity—running can be a peaceful, solitary activity, a time to solve problems and formulate goals. Or perhaps you crave challenges. In that case there is plenty of opportunity to test yourself against other runners or your own times in the many races held during the spring, summer, and fall. Most personalities can find a niche in this sport.

Yet running is not an exercise most people should jump into. Beginners should slowly push their heart rates upward and gradually develop the lower body muscles by alternating between walking and running. But don't translate this as advice to always jog slowly. A slow jog is less effective than a brisk walk; use it only as a transition from walking to running. Then pick up speed to a quick trot. Running at this moderate speed you won't break any records, but you will raise the heart rate and improve your endurance. If that's all you want to do, it's enough.

CROSS-COUNTRY SKIING. As an outdoor activity, cross-country skiing is limited to a very small population. Therefore, I will discuss its indoor version, done on a cross-country ski machine. Like its outdoor ancestor, the indoor machine version gives you a tremendous aerobic workout—sans an occasional chilly glide down a snowy path. All machines have a pair of sliding slats, a tension control that increases resistance, and an upper body attachment that duplicates a skier's poling action. Some machines elevate to simulate skiing uphill. Using all these features, recently inactive people would get a workout that is far too intense for them. I've been exercising on a cross-country ski machine for 10 years and have used the arm attachments once, but I still get an excellent aerobic exercise because I'm using my large leg muscle groups. I prefer to exercise my upper body by lifting weights, which is more precise and manageable.

Cross-country skiing is an excellent nonimpact cardio workout, even for people with knee and back problems. Machines take up relatively little space, adjust easily for other family members, and perform consistently during any season. And without the upper body activity, you can read, scribble notes, or watch TV while you build endurance. For convenience and conditioning, it's hard to beat this exercise.

CYCLING. An exercise that can really get you places, cycling is as effective at conditioning the cardiovascular system as it is fun. With its smooth, low-impact motion, it works the large muscle groups of the lower body, especially the front thighs (quadriceps). Add toe clips and you intensify the workout for the rear thighs (hamstrings). But don't mistake this for its recreational sibling. Many think of cycling as a leisurely activity, a slow, Sunday afternoon ride, with more gliding than peddling. This is not exercise to your heart.

For cycling to challenge your heart, it must be vigorous and continuous. Consider this a problem if you're thinking of riding outdoors. How many people live in a neighborhood where they can ride uninterrupted—no cars, traffic lights, or pedestrians—for over 20 minutes at a time? As for using toe clips outdoors, it's downright dangerous. They take away your ability to ground your feet at a moment's notice. So will earphones. Music may make your trip more enjoyable, but it will also drown out noises you must react to. Still, I won't rule out this mode of cycling for people who live in the right area and love the outdoors. Just don't make it a Tour de France.

To cycle outdoors, you need a three- to five-speed bike with a sturdy frame that can take a pounding. Avoid handle bars that curl under like a ram's horns; they promote poor posture. Handle bars that allow you to sit upright are more comfortable, and they create wind resistance for a more vigorous workout. Another comfort concern is the seat. Riding on the thin, hard seats of many bikes is enough to drive you to an easy chair. Opt for a wide, well-cushioned seat.

Cycling indoors gives you more control. Climate, speed, and resistance are literally at your fingertips, along with other activities such as reading, writing, listening to music, and watching TV.

Whatever you prefer, indoor or outdoor cycling, make it as convenient and comfortable as possible. This isn't survival of the toughest; it's how to become the fittest.

Aerobics. Aerobics is a generic term that describes step aerobics as well as high- and low-impact aerobic dance routines. Workouts are generally designed to work the arms and legs at the same time. As a heart conditioner, it's effective. The legs, supporting and moving the upper body nonstop, create an oxygen demand that raises the heart rate and keeps it up. That also tells you your legs get a good workout. Your arms, however, are another story. Moving them around will do just so much for their muscle tone. Though this in itself isn't a serious problem, the aerobics industry's attempt to solve it is: they have made hand weight and—God save us—leg weight accessories. Do these weights help tone your limbs? No. Do they unnecessarily pound your joints? Yes. Almost universal is the advice that overweight people with ankle, knee, or hip problems lose weight. Holding hand weights and wearing ankle weights, you gain weight. On the surface, it may look like an efficient way to get a better workout; inside your body it is an efficient way to damage your joints. If you want to tone or build your upper body, lift weights—but not while you're doing aerobics.

There are two ways to get an aerobics workout: join a class or buy a home video. An aerobics class gives you camaraderie and social contact. Your home gives you privacy and convenience. If you prefer the home video, however, make sure you choose one that is reputable. Nowadays, every celebrity in America puts out an aerobic exercise video, many of which are neither safe nor effective. Choose one made by a well-respected fitness professional.

Even some reputable videos won't be suitable if they don't match your ability. Many are rated according to difficulty, whether they are high or low impact and the degree to which they are aerobic. In a class, the intensity and duration are out of your control, so enroll in one at your level. That means beginners should join a beginners' class. Never follow an experienced friend to his or her class; you'll set yourself up for a beating—an embarrassing one.

You'll also set yourself up for an injury, a predicament quite common in aerobics. Perhaps it's from choosing the wrong class or video. Perhaps it's the pounding exaggerated by unnecessary weights. Or perhaps it's the poor quality equipment. Step aerobics requires a bench, and all aerobics require good shoes that absorb shock and stabilize your feet.

STAIRCLIMBING. The invention of stairclimbing machines transformed a very old activity into a convenient one-way flight to the highest-intensity aerobic exercise. A good aerobic workout is only one of the selling points of these machines. Depending on where the foot is positioned on the "stair," it can work different leg muscles, and its low-impact motion is safe for those with foot, knee, or back problems.

But stairclimbing may not be the exercise for you. Even on an easy setting, stairclimbing is too taxing for beginners. To become fit you must first form the habit of exercising, a habit based on a feeling of exhilaration and accomplishment, not heart-pounding, sweat-pouring suffering. A stairclimbing machine pushes you. For an experienced exerciser this builds stamina and brings quantum leaps in conditioning. For a beginner, it could just as easily build a bad attitude toward exercise.

ROWING. Like cross-country skiing, rowing has one practical option: doing it on a machine. A rowing machine exercises the upper and lower body with a smooth, low-impact motion that minimizes stress on the ankles, knees, and hips. But it's a total body commitment you must accept; there's no option to uncouple the arm workout from the leg workout as in cross-country skiing. Nor do the legs work as hard. The sitting position relieves them of the upper body's weight, thereby spreading the effort to more muscles throughout the body. This makes rowing a bodywide endurance builder, and with so many muscles working, the cardiovascular system shifts into high gear, quickly improving its own endurance.

SWIMMING. Long touted as the ultimate low-impact exercise, swimming is overrated for several reasons. First, few people have a sizable and preferably indoor pool available to them year-round. Years ago I asked a friend who belonged to a health club why she swam for exercise. "I do it because it's good for my back," she said, "but I usually have to wait to use the pool, and then you're allowed in it for only 15 minutes at a time." And when she did get to swim, there were always "traffic problems." An exercise that's inconvenient is an exercise that's ineffective.

But there's more behind swimming's ineffectiveness than inconvenience. Swimming is mostly an upper body activity that demands little of the legs. As semi-bystanders, the large muscle groups don't need nearly the amount of oxygen they would if they were working hard. Another problem is swimming's unique horizontal position. Coupled with the buoyancy of fat tissue in the water, it decreases the heart and circulatory response relative to the effort expended. The final blow to swimming is the general attitude toward it. Instead of vigorous laps around a pool, many see it as a recreational frolic in the water. If frolicking were exercise, more people would be fit. In short, swimming sounds better to the ear than it does to the heart.

CIRCUIT TRAINING. Circuit training is a version of weight training. It requires a preset arrangement of machines that works different muscles, thereby preventing fatigued muscles from being called on repeatedly. The muscles being worked will go anaerobic—that is, they revert to energy production without oxygen and begin to collect its by-product of lactic acid. After that, it's a matter of time; no muscle can continue to work anaerobically for long and will quickly become exhausted. But by then you will have already moved on to another machine that works different muscles, so you can continue lifting without interruption.

Circuit training is classified as aerobic exercise because it keeps the heart rate up, and that's part of its challenge. Exercising on one machine, say, a stairclimber, is a straightforward task. But you circuit train on at least seven machines, and to keep your heart rate elevated, you must move briskly from one machine to another. Some may find this hectic; others will find it exciting. Everyone, however, must find a spa or gym to do it in unless they're prepared to invest thousands of dollars in equipment.

Good gyms always have an extensive array of equipment. Just make sure that some machines are designated for circuit training so another exerciser can't interrupt your workout by intercepting the one you're about to use. And while you're at it, note the number of circuit machines they do have available. Are there enough to sustain a workout for at least 20 minutes? Some careful research can save you much time and frustration.

Circuit training is a different aerobic exercise. If you have easy access to a well-equipped gym, if the repetition of other aerobic exercises bores you, if you don't mind concentrating a little extra while you exercise, let it be the vehicle to your goals.

ANAEROBIC EXERCISES TO CONDITION SPECIFIC MUSCLES

SIT-UPS (ABDOMINALS). Sit-ups build more endurance than strength. But they are a great toner for your abdomen and a good way to warm up for any workout. The abdominal muscles support the back more than any other muscle group; they are the link between your upper and lower body. If the link is weak, you are vulnerable. The stronger the abdominal muscles, the better they absorb the shock of abrupt movements of your upper and lower body. It's a strength that can save you from considerable back pain.

Always do sit-ups on a padded surface such as a rug with foam padding. There, lie on your back, knees bent, feet flat on the floor, with your hands crossed over your chest or clasped behind your head. Many authorities disapprove of the hands-behind-the-head position; they say it yanks the head and neck forward at too severe an angle. But if the sit-ups are done at a reasonable pace and in a smooth manner, neck jerking won't be a problem.

Another common mistake is to rise up too close to your knees. Many people were taught this style of sit-ups in high school and college. If that's what you learned, unlearn it now. As you rise up, think of your back as creating an angle with the floor; this angle should be between 30 and 40 degrees. Past 40 degrees, the back gets more strain than the abdominal muscles get exercise.

REVERSE TRUNK TWISTS (ABDOMINALS). Even more effective than sit-ups at holding the stomach in are reverse trunk twists. But that washboard look isn't free; you have to earn it by doing a more strenuous exercise that works the side abdominals more than the front. Start by lying flat on your back, arms on the floor (extended perpendicu-

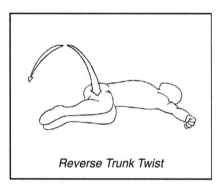

Reverse Trunk Twist

lar to your body), legs raised toward the ceiling (perpendicular to your trunk). Then slowly lower your legs to one side so that they are parallel with your outstretched arms. Next, bring your legs back to their starting point. Again, lower your legs, this time toward the other outstretched hand. Exhale as you lower your legs; inhale as you raise them.

At first you may lack strength and flexibility to fully extend your legs. If you do, start by doing the exercise with your knees bent. This will build your side abdominal muscles, eventually enabling you to do the exercise with outstretched legs. But don't stop here. Challenge yourself by wearing ankle weights while trunk twisting. Your gains will far outweigh your effort.

REVERSE FLIES (UPPER BACK). Primarily an exercise for the upper back, reverse flies also strengthen the back of the neck, the shoulders, and the upper arms. Begin by lying face down on a weight bench with a dumbbell in each hand and your arms extended out from your sides perpendicular to your body. Without bending

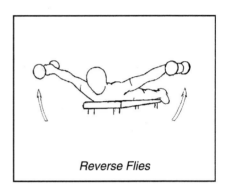

Reverse Flies

your arms, slowly lower your hands to the floor. Then, keeping your arms straight, slowly raise your hands to slightly above your body.

ONE-ARM ROWING (UPPER BACK). One-arm rowing, which requires only one dumbbell and a chair, strengthens the trapezius of the upper and middle back. Bend forward until your back is parallel to the floor. Lean one hand on a bench or the seat of a chair. With the other hand, hold a dumbbell, keeping your arm straight and

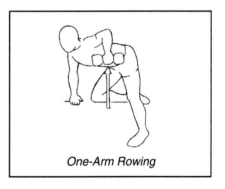

One-Arm Rowing

allowing your shoulder to dip slightly toward the floor. "Row" by slowly pulling the dumbbell up until your elbow is about six inches above your back and slowly return it to the starting position. Proper elbow movement is the key to this exercise. Keep it close to the body as you move the weight upward. If you have trouble finding enough time for workouts, take this exercise to the office and strengthen and invigorate yourself during spare moments.

BACK RAISES (LOWER BACK). Although many exercises reinforce areas around the primary muscle group, a back raise is almost exclusive in its focus on strengthening the lower back. First, lie face down on the floor with your arms at your side. From this position, slowly raise your upper body off the floor high enough to feel significant

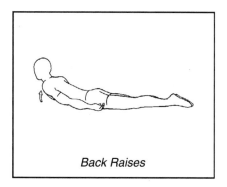

Back Raises

tension in your back muscles. That won't be far, especially without the help of your arms. Back raises don't require weights; therefore, measure your progress by how long you can hold the position and how many you can do.

SUPINE FLIES (CHEST). This exercise strengthens the large pectoral muscles of the chest as well as the deltoid muscles of the front shoulder. Start by lying face up on a weight bench, knees bent, feet on the floor, arms extended straight above your body, each hand holding a dumbbell. Begin the exercise by slowly lowering the dumbbells

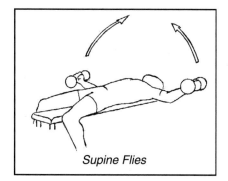

Supine Flies

out to the side until your upper arms are perpendicular to your body. Slowly lift the dumbbells back to their starting position through the same path traced in their descent. Throughout the movement, keep your arms slightly bent at the elbow, inhaling as you lower them, exhaling as you raise them.

BARBELL BENCH PRESS (CHEST). Barbell bench presses condition the pectoral muscles of the chest and, to a lesser extent, the tricep muscles of the arms. Before taking your position, place a barbell on the weight bench rack, making sure the collars are on tight. Then lie on the bench face up, knees bent, feet on the floor. The bar should be directly above your shoulders. Grasp the barbell with your hands slightly more than shoulder width apart, palms facing forward, and slowly lower it to just above your chest. Inhale during

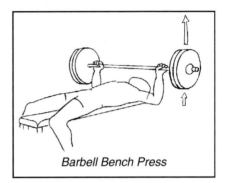

Barbell Bench Press

this movement. Finish by pushing the barbell above your body, exhaling until your arms are straight. Always have a spotter assist you in case you can't get the weight back on the bench rack.

SIDE LIFTS (SHOULDERS). Side lifts strengthen the deltoids, muscles that cap the shoulders. Position yourself by standing, slightly bent forward, hands holding dumbbells just in front of your hips with your palms facing each other. Then, keeping your arms slightly bent, lift the weights out to the side and up, forming an arc, which is completed when you bring the weights over your head. Finish by lowering them slowly along the same arc to the starting

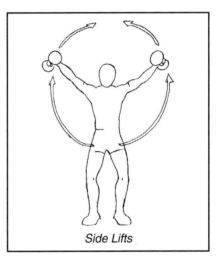

Side Lifts

position. As with most exercises, inhale while you lift, exhale while you lower.

FRONT LIFTS (SHOULDERS). This exercise works your front deltoid shoulder muscles, as well as your upper pectoral chest muscles. To start stand erect, holding dumbbells at hip level, the palm of your hands facing your body. Keeping your arms straight, raise one directly in front of you and continue moving it upward until the dumbbell is higher than your head but not directly above it. Inhale during this movement. Then, exhale as you slowly bring the dumbbell down through the same track you lifted it. Immediately repeat the movement with the other arm; front lifts alternate repetitions between arms.

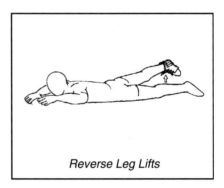

Front Lifts

REVERSE LEG LIFTS (LEGS). Great for conditioning the hamstrings of the rear thigh, reverse leg lifts also tone the buttocks and lower back. Lie on your stomach with your arms folded in front of you. Raise one leg as high as you can; then lower it to where your foot only lightly touches the ground. During this movement concentrate on holding your hip bone against the floor. To raise it makes the exercise easier and defeats its purpose. Reverse leg lifts work one leg at a time—that is, you complete one leg's workout before going to the other. When this exercise becomes too easy, add ankle weights and reduce the number of repetitions.

Reverse Leg Lifts

WEIGHTED LEG EXTENSIONS (LEGS). Leg extensions build the quadriceps, which cover the front of the thighs and stabilize the knee caps. Sit on a table, dresser, or counter top—anything that's sturdy enough to hold your weight and high enough to allow your legs to hang. Slowly extend one leg outward until it is almost straight but not locked and just as slowly lower it to its bent knee starting position. Exercise one leg at a time. Probably your quadriceps are already strong enough to lift ankle weights, so start with them. Eventually, you'll graduate to regular weights suspended by a strap that hangs on your foot.

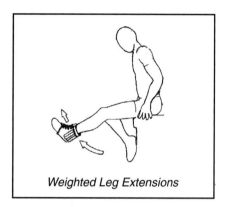

Weighted Leg Extensions

HEEL RAISES (LEGS). The calf muscles lift your weight in this exercise. Stand on a stair with the heels of your feet hanging over the edge. Holding on to something for balance, shift all your weight to one foot and lower that heel as far as possible. This is your starting position. Slowly raise up on your toes; then slowly lower your heels back down to the starting position. Ultimately you'll be able to lower and lift yourself while holding a weight

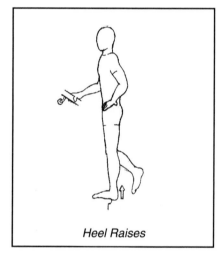

Heel Raises

on the same side as the leg that's exercising. There are many variations of this exercise: some require you to lift yourself from the floor level; others have you exercise both calves at the same time while balancing yourself over the edge of a bench with a barbell across your shoulders. The variation described here is the easiest and most effective.

DUMBBELL CURLS (ARMS). Most of the work of dumbbell curls is done by the bicep muscles of the upper arm, with the inner forearms lending limited assistance. Do this exercise sitting or standing. Hold dumbbells with the palms of your hands facing frontward, arms straight, with upper arms against your side. Then slowly lift the dumbbell to your shoulder, and lower it to its starting position, exhaling as you lift, inhaling as you lower. Throughout the movement your back should be straight and your upper arm against your side. Only your lower arm moves. You can do dumbbell curls one arm at a time or with both arms alternating repetitions. It's a good exercise for those impatient to see their newfound strength in muscle expansion.

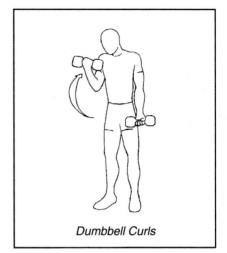

Dumbbell Curls

TRICEP BARBELL CURLS (ARMS). The tricep muscles, which wrap around the side and back of your upper arm, are naturally weak because they are not used for most daily activities; surrounding muscles shelter them from stress by doing work for them. This exercise best isolates them and forces them to work, although they still get a little help from the forearm.

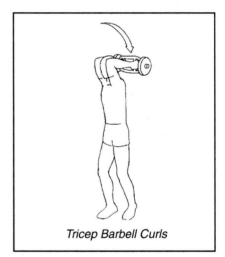

Tricep Barbell Curls

Choose from two starting positions: standing or lying face up on a bench. The rest of the starting position is exactly the same. With your hands six inches apart, palms facing forward, hold a barbell over the top of your head. Without moving your upper arms, slowly lower the barbell behind your head until it is level with the back of your neck. Slowly raise it to its starting position over your head. What isolates the triceps is keeping your upper arms still.

These muscles are probably the weakest part of your arm. By strengthening them you gain a much-needed balance.

KICKBACKS (ARMS). Another tricep strengthener, kickbacks are easy to take to the office because they require only a light dumbbell and the seat of chair. Bend forward until your back is parallel to the floor. Lean one hand on a bench or chair seat and hold a dumbbell with the other. The upper arm of the weighted hand should be against your body and

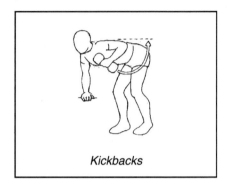

Kickbacks

parallel to the floor with your lower arm bent at a 90-degree angle. From this starting position, slowly straighten your arm as much as possible while keeping your upper arm against your body. Slowly lower the dumbbell to the starting position.

PUSH-UPS (ARMS). Push-ups build the endurance of the shoulder deltoids, chest pectorals, and arm triceps. Assume the starting position by facing the floor, supported only by your straight arms and feet, hands placed where they are comfortable for you. Keeping your body rigid, bend your arms, lowering your chest until your upper arm is parallel to the floor. Once you've pushed yourself back to the starting position, you've completed one standard push-up. Consider that an accomplishment. A standard push-up is a challenge to anyone just starting an exercise program; in fact many beginners won't be able to do even one. If you can't, start with one of two variations. Of these, the better known one is the "modified" push-up, in which you touch the ground with your knees instead of your toes. The other variation is descriptively called the "standing wall push-off." For this exercise, stand with your feet flat and away from the wall and your arms straight, hands against the wall. Then bend your arms until your chest touches the wall and push yourself back to the starting position. The farther your feet are from the wall, the closer these mimic standard push-ups. But remember, these are pseudo push-ups. They are not permanent substitutes for the standards—although some people may want them to be—and they will not help you do more of them. Use them to condition your muscles to the point where you are able to do one standard push-up. Then increase the number of standards you can do by trying to do more of them. Your efforts will be quickly rewarded. As for the other variations, use them to warm up.

These exercises represent a minimum strength-training program for the entire body, and to do all of them would make a very long workout. Limit your workout by exercising different muscle groups on different days: for example, the chest, shoulders, and arms on Mondays and Wednesdays and the legs and back on Tuesdays and Thursdays. Will this build you into an Arnold Schwarzenegger? Not a chance. If that's your goal you're reading the wrong book. It will, however, build strength and endurance.

MATCHING YOUR EXERCISE AND PERSONALITY

Whether aerobic or anaerobic, all the previously mentioned exercises are compatible with the goal of becoming fit. But will they be compatible with your personality? By choosing an exercise, you make a commitment to the future, a commitment you won't be able to honor doing an exercise you absolutely hate. In positive terms, you are more likely to reach your goals doing exercises that mesh with your personality.

Personality is a mixture of genetic and environmental influences, a unique combination of traits represented by the way each person acts and thinks. Yet certain characteristics are common to many people. Figure 4.2 groups these characteristics into combinations that represent various personality types and lists the exercises most likely to agree with them. Probably you'll recognize some of the characteristics under several personality types. Your personality type, however, is the one that contains the most characteristics that belong to you. Read the entire table and identify your personality type. The exercises matched with it may be your best bets to try. Or they may not be.

This figure is not one of the Ten Commandments; it is simply a listing of suggestions for you to contemplate. Personality isn't the only factor to consider in deciding on an exercise. Look at your life. What is going on at work or with your family or even in your mind?

Or perhaps you are interested more in who you want to be, than in who you are now. These are valid considerations.

The point is that you don't have to choose an exercise under your personality type or even one discussed in this chapter. If you feel strongly about doing an exercise, then do it. But do it right. Any exercise handled incorrectly will fail you. There's more to exercise than just running or cycling. There's exercise intensity, frequency, environment—a whole universe of variables that can change it profoundly for you. Learn about them. The more you know, the better your chances of succeeding.

Figure 4.2   **PERSONALITY AND EXERCISE**

Personality Characteristics	Suggested Exercises
Excited by novel situations Enjoy taking risks Easily bored Make quick decisions Extroverted	Group aerobics (if a male) Racewalking Cycling (outdoors) Stairclimbing (with programs) In-line skating *
Enjoy competition Take leadership role Comfortable in social situations Prefer being your own boss Decide after gathering information	Running (5 K, 10 K races) Stairclimbing (challenging intensities) Cycling (competitive) Weight lifting Team sports †
Concerned about what others think Important to "do it yourself" Comfortable in small groups Decide after exhaustive research Perfectionist	Walking Running (middle to long distance) Cycling Rowing Circuit training
Do not mind being alone Frequently tense or anxious Uncomfortable in social situations Not easily bored Introverted	Walking Running (marathons) Cross-country skiing Rowing Swimming

*   *Not discussed in chapter because of safety concerns, but if you don't mind the danger, in-line skating can be an excellent aerobic exercise.*

†   *Not recommended because team sports provide an inadequate workout for the time they take, but you might find an exercise that will help you excel in the sport of your choice.*

COMPARING EXERCISES

	Cardio	Muscular	EXTRA-cising	Conven-ience	Equipment Affordability	Injury Safe
Walking						
Indoors	★★	★	★★★	★★★★	★	★★★★
Outdoors	★★	★	★	★★★	★★★★	★★★★
Running						
Indoors	★★★★	★★	★★★	★★★★	★	★★★
Outdoors	★★★★	★★	★	★★★	★★★★	★★
CC Skiing	★★★★	★★	★★★★	★★★★	★★	★★★★
Cycling						
Indoors	★★★★	★★	★★★★	★★★★	★★	★★★★
Outdoors	★★★★	★★	★	★★	★	★★★
Aerobics	★★★★	★★	★	★★	★★★	★★
Stairclimbing	★★★★	★★	★★★	★★★★	★	★★★
Rowing	★★★	★★	★★	★★★★	★	★★
Swimming	★★	★★	★	★	★★★	★★★★
Circuit Train.	★★★	★★★	★	★★	★	★★★
Wt. Lifting						
Low Rep, High Wt.	★	★★★★	★	★★★★	★★	★★
High Rep, Low Wt.	★	★★★★	★	★★★★	★★	★★★
Push-Ups	★	★★★	★	★★★★	★★★★	★★★
Sit-Ups	★	★★★	★	★★★★	★★★★	★★★★

★ Poor   ★★ Average   ★★★ Good   ★★★★ Excellent

CHAPTER 5

DOING YOUR EXERCISE

"I would rather set my hair on fire than run" [Adele Pace, 1980]. Not only did I make this statement, I lived by it with the fierce resolve of an avowed desk potato. It was an attitude born of experience: a workout with my brother. As a longtime weight lifter and runner, he seemed to be the perfect person to start running with. But a reasonable workout for him was a workout from hell for me. I decided it wasn't going to happen again.

Luckily the experience didn't deafen me. Again and again I kept hearing people who I trusted and admired rave about the great benefits of running. Yet that alone was not enough to get me started again. They were not me. I needed more proof, and using my desk potato skills I got it, reading everything from scientific papers on exercise to magazine articles about the lives and accomplishments of elite runners. It was time and energy well spent. Out of it came the admission that I had been wrong—there was something wonderful about exercise. My goal was to discover what it was. I had a great head start: the right attitude.

Exercising the Right Attitude

Books on fitness seldom address attitude, and it's a serious over-sight. In an age where the mind and body are beginning to be looked at as one, we know that attitude, that preset outlook, can completely change our reality and our reaction to it. It alone can influence the progress of your fitness program or whether you exercise at all. "I hate exercise, but I know I should do it." "Exercise is for some people but not for me." How many times have you heard or said damning statements like these? Why do you hate exercise? Why isn't it for you? Beware of such attitudes; they are not based on logic.

What is based on logic and much research is that a good attitude toward exercise maximizes the chances that it will become a vital part of your life. Think "I can become a bona fide exerciser." See yourself as someone who looks forward to workouts and feels unfulfilled when you miss them. If you can't imagine this (just yet), at least convince yourself that there is something joyous and wonderful about exercise. Then look for it with the right attitude, and you are bound to find it.

Finding the Right Exercise Intensity to Build Your Cardio Fitness

Many bad attitudes toward exercise stem from bad experiences; it felt lousy. Muscle pain and stiffness do not improve the quality of life, and that is exactly what people get when they jump into exercise. It's a common scenario, as predictable as it is avoidable. A nonexerciser's muscles are not conditioned for activity; hence they are unable to use oxygen to produce extra energy. The ability to use more oxygen for energy production comes, over time, from exercising. But people new to exercising have not put this time in when they take their unconditioned muscles for a jog or run. Suddenly their muscles need more energy, so they resort to making it anaerobically. Now these exercisers feel their muscles burning; lactic acid, a by-product of anaerobic energy production, is collecting. The mere presence of lactic acid makes the heart pump faster. That the muscles can't use this extra oxygen makes no difference—the heart must keep pumping more and more. Compounding this problem is the heart's own unfitness. If it were stronger, it could push more blood with each beat. Instead, it must do the same job by beating faster. By now the beginning exerciser is unable to stand the pain and he ends the workout. It's a good thing: his heart is racing too fast.

The Pulse Is the Limit

I call this point the pulse limit. In general it varies depending on your age and sex: aging lowers your limit, and so does, to a small extent, being a woman. Still, no matter what age or which sex you are, you know that you've reached this limit when your muscles burn too much to keep exercising. Your gauge is pain. Scientists use another gauge: oxygen consumption. They measure the maximum volume of oxygen (VO_2 Max) your body can use during the most intense exercise you can tolerate. But both gauges are impractical. Who wants to deal with pain, and who has a private laboratory in which to measure the oxygen content of his or her blood while exercising? Besides, you want to avoid this limit, not reach it.

One gauge you can use to avoid this limit is your heart rate (hence the name "pulse limit"). The point at which your body is using the maximum volume of oxygen is also the point at which your heart is beating fastest. Fortunately, there is a formula based on your age and sex that estimates this limit in heart beats per minute. For a man it's 220 minus his age. For a woman it's 218 minus her age. Both formulas are quick and painless. But an even quicker way to get your limit is to use Figure 5.1. It is a schedule of pulse limits representing averages of various age groups for both men and women, conveniently divided into 15-second time periods (that's how long you should take your pulse). As the formulas indicate, there is not much difference between the pulse limit of a man and a woman. There is also little change in your pulse limit within a ten-year period. Obviously these aren't precise scientific measurements. An estimate, however, is accurate enough to keep you away from the pain that ends so many exercise careers.

The next step is to monitor your actual heart rate, so you can keep it lower than your limit. There are two ways to do this: by taking your pulse manually or by using a pulse meter. To take your

Figure 5.1		PULSE LIMIT		
Age Group	Pulse Limit	45% of Pulse Limit	60% of Pulse Limit	75% of Pulse Limit
20 – 29	49	22	29	37
30 – 39	46	21	28	35
40 – 49	44	20	26	33
50 – 59	41	19	25	31
60 – 69	39	17	23	29

Pulse rates are for a 15-second time period.

pulse manually, press lightly on the area just below your jaw bone, to either side of your throat. What you will feel is the strong pulse of the carotid artery, which runs up both sides of your neck. Never press on both sides of your neck at the same time. Find your pulse on one side only and count it for 15 seconds. If you want to know your heart rate per minute just multiply your count by four.

Taking your pulse this way is easy and accurate, but it does require a break in the action. If you don't want even small breaks in your workout, get a pulse meter. Whichever method you choose, you won't be using it forever. Once you become experienced at gauging your exercise intensity, you won't need to take your pulse; your brain will have learned what your regular workout intensity is, and it will set that intensity for you each time you exercise. Call this your perceived effort and trust it as much as any pulse meter—it's remarkably accurate.

"No Pain, No Gain"—NO WAY

Nevertheless if you're a beginner, you should pay attention to your heart rate. Beginners should stay the farthest from their pulse limit because they have the least conditioning. Figure 5.1 contains heart rates at various percentages of the pulse limit. At 45 percent, you're working at a low intensity, at 60 percent, a moderate intensity, and at 75 percent, a high intensity.

If you're a beginner (see Figure 5.2), work at a low intensity— 45 percent of your pulse limit—during your first week of exercise.

Figure 5.2   **AEROBIC EXERCISE PROGRAM FOR BEGINNER**

	Warm-up	Exercise Duration	Intensity	Cool-down
Week 1	3 minutes	10 minutes	45%	none
Week 2	4 minutes	12 minutes	50%	none
Week 3	4 minutes	15 minutes	55%	none
Week 4	4 minutes	15 minutes	60%	1 minute
Week 5	5 minutes	15 minutes	60%	1 minute
Week 6	5 minutes	15 minutes	60%	1 minute
Week 7	5 minutes	20 minutes	60%	1 minute
Week 8	5 minutes	20 minutes	60%	1 minute

➤ *Exercise intensity is percent of pulse limit per Figure 5.1.*

➤ *If 45 percent intensity is too close to your resting pulse, go to 50 percent but no higher.*

➤ *The 10 percent rule of increasing work by no more than 10 percent in two weeks does not apply to the low levels of intensity involved in preconditioning the muscles of a beginner.*

➤ *Detailed warm-up procedures are discussed in Chapter 6 (Figure 6.3).*

➤ *After completing this eight-week beginner's program follow the sex and age group exercise guidelines in Chapter 15 or 16 (Figure 15.2 or 16.3).*

If this is too close to your resting pulse, increase it to 50 percent, but go no higher. In the second week increase your exercise intensity by five percentage points and move up to 50 percent of your pulse limit. Here you begin to win the battle of the bulge—at 50 percent almost all energy is derived from burning fat, a phase that continues through the third week as you exercise at 55 percent of your pulse limit. Finally, in the fourth week you'll hit 60 percent. Now you are giving your heart a workout intense enough to condition it. It's a milestone you don't have to rush by. Work out at this intensity for an extra two to four weeks, especially if you're over 40 or overweight.

"But," you may say, "what was I doing for the first three weeks if I wasn't conditioning my heart?" Much more than you realize. The odds that people will stick with exercise programs are so low because people are so intent on diving into them head first. By starting gradually, gently introducing your body to exercise, you sway those odds drastically in your favor. This is an approach backed by the American College of Sports Medicine, which is now urging nonexercisers to take part in any exercise or activity even if it falls below the cardiovascular threshold of 60 percent of their pulse limit. They call it "exercise lite." I call it "exercise first"—it's the way every new exerciser or experienced exerciser taking up a new exercise should start. Too many people are prisoners of that silly motto "no pain, no gain." Like troopers they charge ahead. But what they get is much pain and no gain. The human body is not a nail to be hammered; it is a complex organism that has to be shaped and given time to adapt. Gradually intensifying workouts allows for this.

A few weeks of low-intensity aerobic exercise tells your muscles that more is going to be expected of them, and they react by dramatically adapting to accommodate this demand. They become more efficient at using oxygen for producing energy. You'll know when this happens—you won't fatigue or feel the burning of lactic acid as quickly. In short, you won't suffer. This is as nature planned it, because your body evolved for physical activity. But your body needs only a certain kind of physical activity, activity strenuous enough to tax the heart. Suffering need not apply. Ask many of the refugees of exercise and they'll confirm this. They'll tell you how bad exercise felt, how they counted the seconds during each workout, how they got injured. When you tell them that they exercised too hard, that none of the pain was necessary, they become defensive and say something like, "I have a friend who threw himself into exercise and he's still doing it five years later." Maybe so, but that friend is an exception to the rule, a rare bird able to soar where many others have crashed. Admiring someone like this is fine. Modeling your approach to exercise after them is disastrous. Very few exercise habits started this way. There's no shame in going slow—you have the rest of your life.

Fortunately it won't take that long. After one or two months of preconditioning at low to moderate intensity you will be ready to move up. Now you will exercise with your heart rate above 60 percent of your pulse limit, but don't shoot up to 75 percent right away. Such a workout is still too intense. Slowly work your way toward it—if that's where you want to go. Beyond 60 percent you are conditioning your heart and exercising at 75 percent isn't going to condition it much better. Go there only for a personal challenge. (See Figure 5.3 for a sample exercise progression.)

Figure 5.3   SAMPLE PROGRESSION OF AEROBIC EXERCISE

	% of Maximum Heart Rate	Heart Rate Male Age 40 (beats / min.)	Duration of Exercise	Times per Week
Introduction				
Week 1	45%	81	10 min.	3
Week 2	50%	90	12 min.	3
Week 3	55%	99	15 min.	3
Week 4	60%	108	15 min.	3
Cardio Conditioning				
Lifetime	60–75%	108–135	20 min.	3
Elite Training				
Lifetime	75–100%	135–180	Brief intervals	1

Wherever you go, your heart rate must stay there for at least 20 minutes at a time. Your heart needs 20 minutes to become conditioned. It also needs it three times a week. Not that keeping your heart rate up for over 20 minutes isn't better; it is. So is exercising more than three times a week. But at this point it isn't necessary. Remember, what you are trying to do is get into the habit of exercising while you condition your muscles and heart. In the beginning that is quite enough.

Up to this point you probably think that exercise time is the total time you spend exercising—the time between, say, getting on an exercycle and getting off of it—and it's an understandable interpretation. But it's wrong. Strictly defined, exercise time is the time during which your heart rate stays at the target percentage of your pulse limit. When you sit on an exercycle, will your heart rate instantly accelerate to that 65 percent level? No, and you shouldn't try to force it—it's too hard on your exercising muscles. What you must do first is warm up. A warm-up is the antecedent of any workout of moderate or high intensity, and it should specifically match the exercise you plan to do. Don't warm up for a run by riding an exercycle for 5 minutes; that won't warm up the specific muscles used during the workout. Warm up for a run by first jogging slowly. Warm up for cycling by first cycling slowly. A 20-minute workout, as I define exercise time, does not include this warm-up step, and therefore will actually take longer. Factor this extra time into your schedule.

Seven Clues for Recognizing an Exercise Habit

For most people, a workout of moderate intensity will be exercise "home" for the rest of their lives. The rest of your life is a long time. Recently a 40-year-old friend echoed that unsavory—and I might add incorrect—cliché, "After 40 it's all downhill." Exercise not only prevents that, it demonstrates the opposite: after 40 it gets better and easier. As you get older, you can exercise at lower intensities for less time and still maintain the same physical condition. On second thought maybe that cliché is correct. It's easier to walk downhill than it is to climb uphill.

Still some people may want to keep climbing uphill to the next level of intensity above 75 percent of their pulse limit. If that's your goal, first make sure you have the solid foundation of an exercise habit. How do you know if you have one? Look inside yourself. There will be a number of clues.

Clue 1.   When you must miss a regular workout, you're disappointed.

Clue 2.   Things that remind you of your favorite exercise make you look forward to your next workout.

Clue 3.   You enjoy sharing your experiences, feelings, and ideas about exercise with others.

Clue 4.   You see exercise as something that can turn a bad day into a good one.

Clue 5.   You find yourself associating more and more with other exercisers.

Clue 6.   Things related to exercise, such as nutrition, are much more interesting to you now.

Clue 7.   You are tempted to work out when injured or ill.

When you recognize some or all of these clues, you'll know that you have reached one of your most important goals: becoming a life-long exerciser. But don't celebrate that realization too vigorously.

Keeping Your Habit at the Right Level

Ten years ago when I established an exercise habit for the first time, I relished the difference it made in me, physically and emotionally, and I figured if some running is good, more is better. In less than three weeks I increased my mileage from 25 to 45 miles a week. It was one of the biggest mistakes of my life. My knees, not yet conditioned for that many miles, gave out under the stress. It took me years to get them back into running condition.

Let this be a mistake you avoid. First, whenever you increase the intensity or the duration of a workout, give your body time to adjust. Don't think that because you're in good condition you can take it. And second, never increase intensity and duration at the same time.

Some sources recommend increasing intensity or duration no more that 10 percent every week. But no matter how small you think the increase is, the cardinal rule is to give your body enough time to adapt. Except for beginners, who are working at very low intensities, one week is not enough time. I recommend you increase your workout no more than 10 percent every two weeks. With that progression 10 years ago, I would have increased my mileage in three weeks to 30 miles a week instead of 45—a big difference.

Increasing the length of a workout is a straightforward matter. Not so straightforward is the task of increasing exercise intensity. Do not use time versus distance as a gauge. If you run, for example, you could intensify a workout by running faster—either the same distance in less time or a longer distance in the same time. But while this computes to 10 percent faster on paper, your heart may not agree. The best way to form an exercise habit—as I stated earlier in this chapter—is to use your heart rate as the gauge of your exercise intensity. Therefore it makes sense that increases in intensity should be measured by heart rate.

The safest way to turn up exercise intensity is to do it intermittently throughout a workout. Introduce short periods of higher intensity by sandwiching them between periods of normal intensity and then gradually lengthening them. These mini-exposures to higher intensity help your body adapt. It's an approach that works with any aerobic exercise.

Of course even the best plans don't always work. Everyone is different. If you've gradually introduced an intensity increase to your workouts and you still feel tired and sore, cut back. Sometimes there's more than a workout involved, perhaps some added stress from work or a family crisis. Sometimes there won't seem to be any reason. Be patient. The gradual approach can take you just about anywhere.

TECHNIQUES TO BUILD YOUR MUSCULAR STRENGTH AND ENDURANCE

I began weight lifting to build the "overcooked linguini" arms my brother often teased me about. His assessment was as accurate as it was creative. As a person genetically disposed to a slight frame and small muscles, my entire upper body—arms, shoulders, chest, and back—were shockingly weak. More aerobic exercise wasn't the answer. I had already conditioned my cardiovascular system and lower body muscles. What I needed was strength in my upper body. That meant a voyage into the sea of anaerobic exercise, which, unlike my steady and continuous aerobic exercise, consisted of waves of strenuous exercise broken up by periodic rests. Over the next few years I lifted weights two or three times a week, and even though the workouts were never long, my progress was impressive. As I made the weights I lifted heavier and heavier, my strength grew. No longer did I have linguini arms. But like many weight lifters I didn't recognize the significance of my increased strength. Then I joined the Army Reserves.

As a member of the Army Reserves, I had to take the Army Physical Fitness Test. One of its requirements is to do 13 push-ups. I was able to do 18. But I was shocked that I could do any—until then I had never done a push-up in my life.

Before I took the test, I quickly warmed up with a short jog. It was all I had time to do. As with aerobic exercise, anaerobic exercise calls for a warm-up beforehand. This warm-up, however, has not one, but two phases: first a general overall body warm-up, followed by a more specific warm-up to prepare the muscles you will be using. For the general warm-up, any light aerobic exercise will do. For the specific warm-up, you must lightly exercise the muscle groups to be used during the workout by doing one exercise with a lighter than usual weight for each muscle group. Even though this doesn't take too long, it may seem like warm-up overkill. But you are subjecting your muscles to intense and unusual stress, and they must be prepared.

Use the Right Weight-Lifting Techniques

After properly warming up your muscles, make sure your mind is prepared too. An aerobic workout usually places no real demand on the mind; it is free to stray wherever it pleases. But while weight lifting, your mind must be fixed on your form—slowly moving the weight along the full range of motion required by the exercise. This isn't for appearances. Good form guards against injury and guides your power where it belongs—in your lifts.

Start with your posture. When lifting weights, always keep your back straight, with your shoulders slightly back. For many people holding this position will be as much of a challenge as the exercise itself; they don't even have good posture when sitting or walking around, let alone when they lift weights. If this is you, rise to the occasion by straightening up; it maximizes the stability of your spine, which helps to bear the extra weight.

For those who choose not to rely on their posture, there are weight-lifting belts. Worn snugly, the belt supports your lower back when you lift weights your body isn't used to. It's a form of insurance many weight lifters use. Weight lifters also frequently wear gloves to prevent the build-up of callouses and to give them a better grip. A good grip is indispensable when lifting heavy weights and will help you to maintain proper form during the difficult final repetitions.

Breathing is also an integral part of good form. Haphazard huffing and puffing just divert your energy from the exercise. Always breathe smoothly throughout the motion of the exercise, exhaling while lifting, inhaling while returning to the starting position. Avoid holding your breath while straining; this causes a big increase in blood pressure.

In fact your entire workout should be smooth, from picking up the weights and lifting them through the motion, to putting them down. Never yank the weights. This is cheating, and you don't get away with it. While a jerky motion does nothing to build strength and endurance, it can cause injuries such as torn muscles and inflamed tendons. So can dropping weights. Such a quick release imitates a jerky motion, with all its unnatural forces.

These are not the only unnatural forces you need to avoid. Another is the force of a weight that you no longer have the strength to lift. In one respect you want this. The final repetitions before exhaustion promote the most growth. But not if you're doing a bench press alone. Then the situation can be life threatening— unless you use a spotter. A spotter is another person, preferably another weight lifter, who is able to assist you with your exercise. Then you can flirt with exhaustion during your bench press. Otherwise don't do them. Good technique is safe technique.

Finally, proper weight lifting technique warrants a particular order of business. When you exercise, always work the torso muscles—chest, back, shoulders, and midsection—first. No matter what muscle group you work on, your arms must always hold the weights. Tire them first and you limit what your torso can do.

The Reasons for Repetitions and Intervals

With form and safety in mind, let's review some basic weight-lifting lingo. Strength is the product of stressing a muscle with a weight. One way to stress a muscle is to increase the weight it must move. After each increase, the weight will feel heavy, but several workouts later, they will begin to feel lighter. The weight didn't change, your strength did.

But how much weight you lift isn't the only variable in a workout. How many repetitions (reps) you are able to do also varies. A repetition is one complete motion of an exercise from the starting point through the entire motion back to the starting point. To build strength, use heavy enough weights to limit the number of reps you can do. To build endurance, use lighter weights so you can do more reps (see Figure 5.4).

Figure 5.4 **REP RULES**

Weights allowing:

3 – 10 repetitions	Builds strength and size
10 – 15 repetitions	Builds strength, size and endurance
15 – 25 repetitions	Builds endurance
25 – over repetitions	Wastes time

Knowing how much weight will put you in one category or the other requires experimentation. It also requires that you exercise care so you won't be overwhelmed by postworkout soreness or perhaps an injury. Therefore start light. That refers not only to the weights you lift but also to your rest intervals between sets, a set being a group of repetitions for a specific exercise.

Without enough rest between sets, your muscles stay fatigued—the weights feel heavier than they actually are, and you end up exhausted. Rest intervals are intended to let your heart rate return to normal. During your first workouts that should take between 60 and 120 seconds. Resting longer than 120 seconds allows your muscles to cool, and cool muscles forebode injury. When you are more experienced, you can decrease your rest interval to between 30 and 60 seconds. This represents an intensification of your exercise without increasing the weight or the number of sets, and it allows you to build more strength or endurance in *less* time.

Getting Started with a Weight-Lifting Program

Let your first week of lifting weights be an introduction. Don't start out hoisting heavy weights. Instead use only very light weights and do one set of 30 repetitions for each exercise. Referred to as shadow lifting, this technique focuses on how and where you move the weights, not on how much weight you move. Does this sound too simplistic? You'd be surprised how many weight lifters use bad form because they never gave their mind and muscles a chance to learn the exercises without the burden of heavy weight.

Week 2 is an exploratory week, when you experiment with heavier weights to find ones that you can lift 20 to 25 times in a set. If you can do more than 25 reps with good form, the weight is too light. If your form breaks down before you reach 20 reps, the weight is too heavy. Give yourself a couple of workouts to find what weights you can lift only 20 to 25 times for each exercise; then add a second set of repetitions preceded by a 60-second rest. You'll probably be able to do more repetitions in the first set than you can in the second. This is entirely normal. So is some minor soreness or stiffness the next morning. But don't resent this passing discomfort; it's proof that you have conditioned your muscles for the demands of week 3.

In week 3, increase the weights so you can lift them only 10 to 15 times and drop back to one set. When you do two sets, you gain 80 percent of your strength in the first and 20 percent in the second, so passing on the second won't impede much progress. If you have time and want that last 20 percent of strength, do the second set after a 60-second rest.

Week 3's lifting range of 10 to 15 repetitions falls between the power building range of 3 to 10 repetitions and the endurance range of 15 to 25 repetitions. That makes it an all-purpose range that builds size and strength as well as endurance. Stay in this lifting range as long as you like, but don't allow yourself to stagnate. As your strength grows, which it quickly will in the beginning, the weights will begin to feel too light, and you'll be able to do more than 15 repetitions. The intensity of your workout will decrease. When this first happens, note it. Then go through one more workout with those weights, increasing them the workout after that so you can again do only 10 to 15 repetitions. (See Figure 5.5 for a summary of how to begin a program of weight lifting.)

Exercising at the right intensity, you can do the same aerobic workout every day. This is not so with weight lifting. After a workout, each muscle group exercised should be rested between 48 and 72 hours. Exactly how much recovery time you need depends on your age and, of course, the condition of your muscles. As you get older, your recovery time will lengthen, a fact you might at first take

Figure 5.5   **ANAEROBIC EXERCISE (Weight Lifting)**

	Poundage	Number of Sets	Objectives
Week 1, Shadow Lifting			
Session 1	Ultra light (3–5 lb)	1	Introduction
Session 2	Ultra light (3–5 lb)	1	
Week 2, Experimenting			
Session 1	Light enough to be	1	Shape workouts
Session 2	able to do 20–25 reps	2*	Precondition muscles
Week 3, Establishing			
Session 1	Heavy enough to	1	Build strength
Session 2	allow only 10–15 reps	2*	Build size
			Build endurance

* Rest 60 to 120 seconds between sets.

as a sign that the road of life does lead you downhill after 40. But age has its advantages too. Someone over age 50 can do one-third fewer sets of exercises for the same results as someone younger. In general, people who lift weights look for one of two results: improved strength and endurance or maintenance of strength and endurance. If you want to *improve* your strength and endurance, immediately follow each recovery period with another workout of those muscles. This means exercising the same muscle groups two or three times a week. If you want only to *maintain* your strength and endurance, exercise just once a week, no matter what age group you're in.

Of course the initial goal of all new weight lifters is to improve their strength. But eventually strength gains will slow and then plateau. At this point take a hard look at your workouts. From here, where do you want to go? Do you want to climb another step up the ladder of strength, or do you want to maintain what you have?

To go higher you must power lift or revamp your program. Revamp your program by changing the exercises you do, adding new ones, deleting old ones. The number of exercises for each muscle group can stay the same. This kind of experimentation is fun, and it enables you to be more flexible with your workouts as you expand your knowledge about weight lifting. How can this make you stronger? It tricks your muscles. A muscle that is familiar with an exercise can do it with less effort—it has learned it well and knows how to get the job done easiest. Switch to another exercise and it won't know how to take a shortcut (just yet anyway). Therefore a new exercise is more work for your muscles, and more work builds more strength. As for power lifting, here you enter the domain of weights you can lift only 3 to 10 times. Lifting such heavy weights requires great concentration on form. This is exercise at its most intense. Do it only with a clear goal in mind.

By building muscular strength and endurance through weight lifting, you move closer to your goal of total fitness. But weight lifting builds muscles that are inelastic. Missing in them is flexibility. Flexibility is the most neglected aspect of muscular fitness; few exercisers realize how important it is. Yet flexibility belongs in every exercise program—in fact it's so important, the entire next chapter is devoted to it.

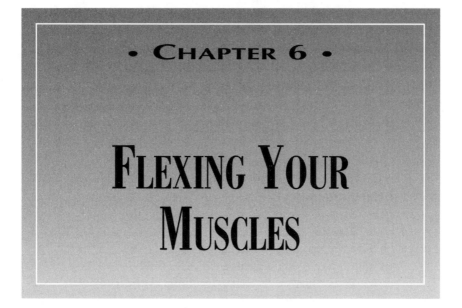

CHAPTER 6

FLEXING YOUR MUSCLES

What would you think if a friend commented that his boss was inflexible? Would you think that the boss is physically stiff, unable to bend easily or reach for things? No, you would think that the boss is stubborn, with a few other rude adjectives added to round out the description of his general personality problem. It's a normal interpretation. Given the lack of emphasis on physical flexibility, the word "flexible," when applied to people, has come to rely on other definitions, and it signals that something must be done to change our attitudes.

Flexibility is more than just a special trait needed by ballerinas and gymnasts; it's an integral part of muscular fitness. But few people seem to know it. Even exercisers who obviously demonstrate a sincere concern about their bodies relegate flexibility to a dusty corner of their itineraries and never seem to get to it. They don't realize that without it, their physical and mental fitness isn't complete.

REGAIN YOUR YOUTHFUL LOOK WITH INCREASED FLEXIBILITY

A flexible person has the ability to move each part of his or her body through its full range of motion. Some movements involve just one joint and its related muscles. Other movements involve several joints. All these movements we should be able to do painlessly and without injury, but many of us can't.

Flexibility is not an attribute of infancy or very early child-hood—babies and young children aren't naturally "double jointed." It's an ability that slowly grows with us. At our most flexible, we are somewhere between adolescence and early adulthood, but the limberness is short-lived, and it gradually leaves as we get older.

How much leaves us depends on how much stretching we do. That is not to say, however, that stretching is the only way to be flexible. Some people are naturally endowed with more flexibility because of a genetic trait, and women tend to be more flexible because of their hormones. But too much flexibility is as bad as too little, as the Army found out when it noticed that the recruits most often injured fell into two groups: those with too little flexibility and those with too much. The problem of too much flexibility is rare, though. Most of us, women included, stand rigidly on the other side of the fence.

If you're beginning to feel old and stiff, wondering just how inflexible you really are, find out by measuring your flexibility with the yardstick test. Sit on the floor with your feet 8 inches apart and place a yardstick between your legs, lining it up so that the 15-inch mark is even with your feet (no shoes) and the higher inch marks are beyond them. Then, bending at the hips, with your back as straight as possible, lean forward as far as you can and mark the yardstick where you are able to reach. Now you know the inches you can reach. Convert them into an estimated flexibility rating by referring to the table in Figure 6.1. Notice the word "estimated." It tells that the table yields only estimates because its conversion factors are not being adjusted for age or sex. Therefore if you are over 40, increase your rating by one standing, moving yourself, for example, from a poor rating up to an average rating.

Figure 6.1	THE YARDSTICK TEST
Flexibility Rating	**Reaching Point**
Superior	22 inches and above
Above average	18 – 21 inches
Average	14 – 18 inches
Poor	11 – 13 inches
Avoid sudden movements	Below 11 inches

Don't despair if your flexibility rating is "poor" or below—your body is very forgiving. With just a little stretching it springs to life, as if it were never neglected. Even beyond the age of 50, you have the potential to regain most of your flexibility.

Lack of flexibility is one of the hallmarks of aging. Everyone can picture the little old lady who totters stiff-leggedly across the street with the help of a Boy Scout, or the old man, bent over, cane in hand, who shuffles slowly toward his destination. Is their condition your destination when you get old? It depends on your attitude. I always think that the old people who drive motorized "wheelchairs" around the supermarket have given up. Somehow they made it into the store by using their legs—they're not crippled—but alas they *are* old and can't possibly make it around the supermarket if there's a wheelchair to carry them. They didn't give up when they reached the supermarket; though they gave up years ago. Loss of flexibility has more to do with how little your body moves than it does with how old your body is.

Flexibility keeps you looking and feeling young. It makes activities an inflexible person wouldn't even try feel easy. You can easily reach the bridge token that rolled under the passenger seat, or help a friend remove her sweater in a cramped restaurant, or remove a splinter from the bottom of your own foot. And these are only a few of the countless tasks that inflexible people must grind and strain through every day. Inflexibility wastes their time and energy.

Flexible Muscles Relax You

Inflexibility also keeps the muscles much too tense. By exerting unnatural forces on the skeletal system, chronically tense muscles cause many problems, including back pain, muscle pulls, joint dislocations, and poor posture. Remember the stooped old man? Flexible muscles are relaxed muscles.

Throughout this book I remind you that the mind and body function as one unit. It's widely known that aerobic exercise decreases anxiety. What isn't so well known is the effect relaxed muscles have on the brain. The brain is constantly monitoring all functions of the body, including muscular tension. If the tension is low, the brain concludes that there is no threat; therefore it has nothing to worry about and you feel calm. High muscle tension sends the opposite message to the brain, and it reacts by giving you a feeling of anxiety. Something is wrong here, it tells you. This relationship between muscle tension and anxiety is used in biofeedback therapy where an electrode taped over a muscle converts the tension it reads into noise. The more noise, the higher the level of tension. Hearing the noise, the participant then concentrates on decreasing it by relaxing his muscles, which, in turn, relaxes his mind. But you don't need expensive noise-making equipment to calm down. By increasing your flexibility, you not only relax your muscles; you smooth out your movements—a double message that the brain translates into a calm emotional outlook. Gone is the anxiety that so cripples your mental sharpness and creativity.

Protect Yourself from Injury

With relaxed muscles you have another advantage: your chances of getting injured are lower. How many times have you heard about the person who hurt his neck or wrenched his back by assuming an unusual position—not a violent or jerking movement, just a position the body isn't used to? It happens too often. Besides the pain, the expensive visits to doctors, and the days missed at work, there is the immense aggravation these injuries bring. "When my back was injured last summer, nobody could even talk to me. I was that short-fused," a business acquaintance once said to me. What is most aggravating is that the injuries are completely avoidable. They just don't happen to flexible people.

A car accident proved it to me. Going 50 miles an hour, the car I was driving hit an oil slick. It spun clockwise, hit a divider, rebounded into a counterclockwise spin, hit the divider again, and finally stopped in the middle of the road. The car was totaled. But I walked away without a scratch—or any of the aches and pains that so often show up later. Much of the credit goes to the seat belt I was wearing. The rest goes to my flexibility. Four months earlier, a friend who teaches karate had started me on a total body flexibility program. Without it, the violence of the wreck would have surely torn some muscles and injured my neck.

But you don't need a violent, twisting movement to hurt your lower back. In fact you don't need any movement. What causes this, the most common and costly injury in the United States, are tight hamstrings, buttock, and lower back muscles. Together the tight muscles conspire against weak abdominals. It becomes a nasty game of tug-of-war won by the tight muscles, and over time their imbalanced pull injures the spine causing intermittent or chronic pain. Relaxing the tight muscles and strengthening the abdominals frees the spine from those damaging forces. Of all the different kinds of injuries you can get, those caused by muscular tightness are the most avoidable. Flexible muscles can prevent a back injury and the gnawing pain that accompanies it; they can also guard other areas of the body vulnerable to chronic muscle imbalances.

Flexibility is a natural treatment for pain, even when there is no injury. Muscle soreness from exercise, for example, is not an injury; it's the slight breakdown and rebuilding of muscle, a healthy process that makes the muscle stronger than before. Flexible muscles rebuild with less pain and they grow stronger and more injury resistant than they would without flexibility. All this flexibility adds to the dividend paid on your exercise investment.

PERFORMANCE STRETCHING PREPARES YOUR MUSCLES FOR ACTIVITY

Muscles aren't naturally flexible; they tend, instead, to grow too short and tight. To counter this tendency you must stretch muscles. But what exactly does stretching a muscle mean? Does it mean stretching the actual cells or increasing the distance between cells? By the sound of it, either one could apply; yet neither does.

Muscle is made of muscle cells *and* connective tissue. The connective tissue, a "plastic wrap"–like substance, wraps groups of muscle cells into bundles and rewraps those bundles into groups of bundles, forming throughout the muscle a network of "plastic wrap" layers that fuse into a thicker cordlike band as the muscle tapers. These bands, which connect muscle to bone, are called tendons. I described the connective tissue for a reason: when you stretch to increase flexibility, you stretch the connective tissue—the "plastic wrap"—around and between muscle fibers, not the muscle itself. When the connective tissue tears, it violently takes the muscle along, damaging its cells too. If there is no muscle damage, the tear is to a tendon or ligament. All these injuries are well known in the sports world, where it is accepted that the difference between winning and injury is sometimes stretching. Few, if any, competitive athletes neglect stretching. Unfortunately stretching will not protect ligaments, the connectors between two bones. A stretched ligament is a sprain. Hence, there is more to stretching than just trying to stretch your whole body: you have to know what to stretch and how to stretch it.

Muscle fibers and connective tissue don't always work together. Suppose, for example, you move quickly or even violently, stretching a muscle. The nerve fibers that monitor the muscle length will detect a drastic change and order a contraction to right things by shortening the muscle again, a reflex response aimed at preventing overstretching and tears. But it also prevents the connective tissue from stretching. Quick movements don't work.

Yet a generation ago, this was exactly how we did stretch, bouncing in different positions as if our bodies were made of remarkable rubber bands that never break. Referred to as ballistic stretching, this technique is pointless and dangerous. When you bounce touching your toes, your hamstrings contract. At best nothing is accomplished because the contraction or shortening of the muscle prevents the connective tissue from stretching; at worst you can overstretch a tendon or tear a muscle. I can still remember Rocky Balboa in the first *Rocky* bouncing in and out of stretches. It's a miracle he was fit to fight.

Today's stretching technique respects the actual make up of muscle and how it behaves—the reflex safety mechanism and the relationship between muscle fiber and connective tissue. For effective stretching follow my six-step technique.

1. Slowly enter into a stretch position.

2. Maximum stretch to mild discomfort only.

3. Restrict stretch to normal range of motion.

4. Breathe in a relaxed manner.

5. Hold stretch 10 to 15 seconds (performance stretching) or over 30 seconds (developmental stretching).

6. Slowly exit from a stretch position.

At first you may have to concentrate on moving *slowly* into the stretching position; the outdated technique of bouncing is an accepted habit that must be pried away from your psyche with the crowbar of logic. I still see runners at local races bouncing up and down, this way and that way. They think they're stretching. I think they would perform better if they really stretched.

Next, don't stretch into the painful zone. Pain is a negative signal: it may mean that you are causing your muscle to contract reflexively, thus denying its connective tissue a chance to stretch or that you are tearing a muscle or overstretching a tendon. What you should feel at the maximum point of your stretch is a mild discomfort only. Most people new to stretching aren't quite sure where this point is or how mild discomfort feels. But as you establish your stretching routine, you will develop a feel for what is safe and what is not.

Any stretching routine should increase your range of motion, but only to the limit of how your body was meant to move. A split, with all its drama, may seem like a breach of this rule, yet it is merely an extreme of the normal range. Other movements aren't. The knee, for example, was not meant to bend sideways. Nor was the neck and back meant to bend enough to allow the head to touch the buttocks. Figure 6.2 illustrates safe, effective stretching positions. Stick with these and avoid bizarre and unhealthy stretches concocted by some so-called stretching experts.

Figure 6.2   *Stretches*

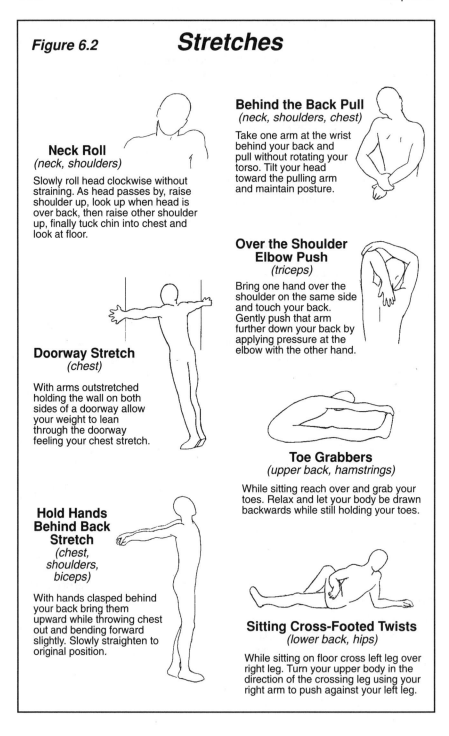

Neck Roll
(neck, shoulders)

Slowly roll head clockwise without straining. As head passes by, raise shoulder up, look up when head is over back, then raise other shoulder up, finally tuck chin into chest and look at floor.

Doorway Stretch
(chest)

With arms outstretched holding the wall on both sides of a doorway allow your weight to lean through the doorway feeling your chest stretch.

Hold Hands Behind Back Stretch
(chest, shoulders, biceps)

With hands clasped behind your back bring them upward while throwing chest out and bending forward slightly. Slowly straighten to original position.

Behind the Back Pull
(neck, shoulders, chest)

Take one arm at the wrist behind your back and pull without rotating your torso. Tilt your head toward the pulling arm and maintain posture.

Over the Shoulder Elbow Push
(triceps)

Bring one hand over the shoulder on the same side and touch your back. Gently push that arm further down your back by applying pressure at the elbow with the other hand.

Toe Grabbers
(upper back, hamstrings)

While sitting reach over and grab your toes. Relax and let your body be drawn backwards while still holding your toes.

Sitting Cross-Footed Twists
(lower back, hips)

While sitting on floor cross left leg over right leg. Turn your upper body in the direction of the crossing leg using your right arm to push against your left leg.

Figure 6.2 (continued).

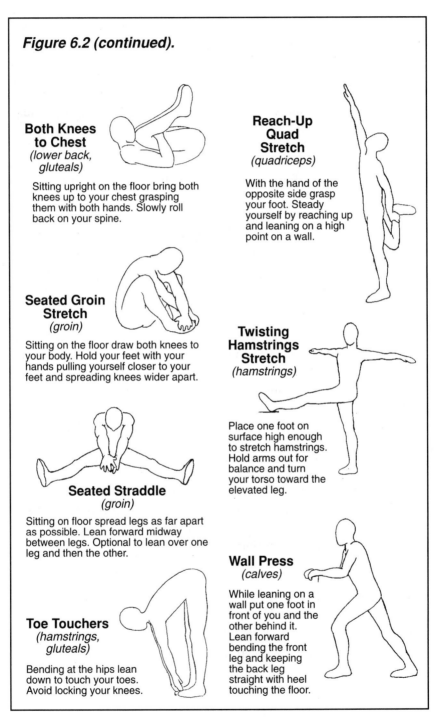

Both Knees to Chest
(lower back, gluteals)

Sitting upright on the floor bring both knees up to your chest grasping them with both hands. Slowly roll back on your spine.

Seated Groin Stretch
(groin)

Sitting on the floor draw both knees to your body. Hold your feet with your hands pulling yourself closer to your feet and spreading knees wider apart.

Seated Straddle
(groin)

Sitting on floor spread legs as far apart as possible. Lean forward midway between legs. Optional to lean over one leg and then the other.

Toe Touchers
(hamstrings, gluteals)

Bending at the hips lean down to touch your toes. Avoid locking your knees.

Reach-Up Quad Stretch
(quadriceps)

With the hand of the opposite side grasp your foot. Steady yourself by reaching up and leaning on a high point on a wall.

Twisting Hamstrings Stretch
(hamstrings)

Place one foot on surface high enough to stretch hamstrings. Hold arms out for balance and turn your torso toward the elevated leg.

Wall Press
(calves)

While leaning on a wall put one foot in front of you and the other behind it. Lean forward bending the front leg and keeping the back leg straight with heel touching the floor.

Working with a friend you can get more out of some stretches. To stretch your hamstrings, for example, sit on the floor with your feet straight out in front of you and have a friend help you bend toward your feet by pushing gently on your back. The help allows you to stay more relaxed, and therefore get a longer stretch. Any stretch that requires a difficult posture is better done with help. But don't let your helper set your limits. Someone else cannot feel what you feel and has no way of knowing if you are being pushed too far. Always tell your helper when to stop. Stretching with a friend can be great fun; just remember that it is the person being stretched who calls the shots.

Breathing is another aspect of stretching where normal is best. Some "experts" tell you precisely when to breathe in and out. This is overkill. What is important is that you keep breathing relaxed and slow. By breathing in a relaxed and natural manner, you get the most out of a stretch. Inhaling and exhaling at specific times applies to weight lifting, where blood pressure control is necessary, not to stretching.

How long you hold a stretch depends on your purpose. If your goal is to maintain your flexibility or prepare your muscles, specifically their connective tissue, for activity, you should do *performance stretching*. If you want to increase your flexibility, permanently changing the length of the connective tissue, you should do *developmental stretching*. A performance stretch is held for 10 to 15 seconds, a developmental stretch for over 30 seconds. Choosing between the two, you'll obviously get what you stretch for.

Of the two kinds of stretching, performance stretching is the more familiar one. If asked, however, most exercisers will identify it as a warm-up. But performance stretching is only a part of the process that prepares the muscles, joints, and cardiovascular system for exercise. With warming-up there is more involved.

THE VITAL ROLE OF WARMING-UP AND COOLING-DOWN

Warming-up is something exercisers just don't have the time for—a luxury in one opinion, a waste in another. Either opinion is costly. Not only does it denigrate the importance of warm-ups, it overestimates the time needed to do them.

Warm-ups are not an option to choose whenever time permits. Do professional athletes ever compete without first warming up? The answer is no—not if they're sane. "But," you may say, "they are competing in world-class events. I am exercising in my den." True, you are not on their level, but neither do you need to warm up as they do. A professional athlete warms up for quite a long time— over 30 minutes. To him it's a ritual that prepares both his body and his mind—it's part of his workday and part of his success.

For you a much shorter and simpler warm-up will accomplish just as much: it will ensure your exercise success. Think of each workout as a personal competition, without the other competitors or the time clocks that record to a hundredth of a second. Then think of what you are competing with: your body. What a marvelous machine it is. But marvelous does not mean bionic; it's unreasonable to push it from rest to vigorous exercise in ten seconds, especially if you work out in the morning. Although there are advantages to morning exercise, one disadvantage is that your body is stone cold at the time, and it must be warmed up even more to prevent the injuries of negligence: the pulls, tears, and sprains, the chronic irritations that mysteriously turn into major inflammations, and worst of all, the heart attack. Notice I said you need to warm up *more* in the morning. By exercising at night you don't avoid this step. The body may be warmer then, but it's still cold in the sense of being ready for exercise.

Warming-up is a four-step process with the fourth step, a mild form of your exercise, being the most likely one to be done by non-professional exercisers. The other three steps are usually neglected.

Step 1 is a light form of aerobic exercise. For 1 or 2 minutes cycle or jog in place to give your heart a wake-up call that prepares it for action. Your heart will take it from there. Wide awake, it pumps more blood to the muscles, waking them up as well.

Step 2 consists of rotational movements. Begin with your head, gently rolling it for three rotations clockwise and three counter-clockwise. Your shoulders are next. Their rotation is a shrug, which continues forward then down, behind, and back up again. Moving on to the pelvis, you might be reminded of a childhood activity. Remember hoola hoops? Pretend you are moving a small hoola hoop around your hips by gently pushing your pelvis forward, sideways, back, and sideways again. Then go still further down to the knees, those ever-fragile joints. Bending them slightly, rotate them in a small circle, straightening them, though not completely for the back part of the rotation. Finally, flex your ankles by gently rotating your foot. Again, rotate each joint three times clockwise and three times counterclockwise. These circular movements, which take only about a minute and a half, spur the joints to lubricate themselves so that they are literally oiled and ready for action.

The third step to warming up is performance stretching. Here you stretch all areas of the body—the neck and shoulders, the back and chest, the abdomen and hips, and the upper and lower legs. Using the six-step stretching method, you will need 2 to 3 minutes for these.

The last step is lightly doing the exercise you are warming up for. Most exercisers start their workout this way and include the few minutes it takes in their overall exercise time. Therefore, I do not add those minutes to your warm-up time.

If you use the maximum time allotted for the first three steps, you'll spend $6\frac{1}{2}$ minutes warming up—very little time when you consider what it does for your mind and body. Make warm-ups part of your exercise routine, even if you are a beginner and your workouts are really too short and easy to require them. Entrench the habit at the onset of your fitness program. After a while warm-ups will become so second nature, you won't even realize that you are doing them. (See Figure 6.3 for a summary of warming up.)

Figure 6.3	**WARMING UP**
Heart	Engage in mellow aerobic exercise to get your heart pumping a little harder. Jog in place or exercycle slowly (1 to 2 minutes).
Joints	Slowly rotate around neck, shoulder, pelvis, knee and ankle joints three times clockwise, three times counterclockwise ($1\frac{1}{2}$ minutes).
Stretch	Do performance stretching for major muscle groups (2 to 3 minutes). 1. Slowly enter into stretch position. 2. Maximum stretch is to mild discomfort. 3. Restrict stretch to normal range of motion. 4. Breathe in a relaxed manner. 5. Hold stretch for 10 to 15 seconds. 6. Slowly exit from stretch position.
Exercise	Very slowly begin your chosen exercise (5 minutes).

The flip side of warming-up is cooling-down. During vigorous exercise your heart beats faster to send more oxygen-rich blood to the working muscles. The muscles take in the blood, use its oxygen, and then as part of the normal effort of exercise, contract, squeezing the blood out and back to the heart. The back-and-forth rush of blood raises the blood pressure.

When you stop exercising suddenly, your blood, which momentarily keeps arriving from the heart in greater quantities, pools in the muscles because they are no longer contracting to squeeze it out. Now at least half the process that was keeping the blood pressure higher has stopped, with the other half dwindling quickly as the heart rate returns to normal. It's a dangerous situation. While the blood pools and the blood pressure plummets, there is not enough blood to go around, and the brain and heart starve. Not enough blood to the brain can cause fainting. Not enough blood to the heart can cause arrhythmia, a disruption of its normal heart beat. These maladies can happen with a healthy brain and heart. If they are not so healthy, having arteries with constrictions, you could have a heart attack or stroke. Those are pretty serious consequences that can be avoided by simply cooling down after a workout. Yet the number of exercisers who bother to cool down falls well short of the already small number who warm up. If you often get light-headed after standing from a stooped position, you are particularly at risk for having postworkout problems. But one principle applies to everybody: the harder you work out, the more important it is to cool down.

Speaking as one person prone to such dizziness, I take special precautions after very hard workouts. Whenever I run a race, I have someone "collect" me at the finish line and keep me walking at a decent pace. Otherwise I might stop cold, my exhaustion overruling all judgment and the knowledge that I must cool down. Normal workouts, of course, shouldn't leave you in this condition. They will, however, leave you vulnerable if you don't cool down.

To cool down, keep your body moving for 3 or 4 minutes; the continued muscle contractions will prevent the blood from pooling, giving your body the time it needs to stabilize blood pressure. Meanwhile, you enjoy some light activity that leaves you feeling better for the rest of the day.

I like to follow my cool-down with some stretching while my muscles are still warm. It's a short step down from cooling off—you are still moving your muscles, though more passively than, say, walking, and at this time, it most effectively soothes and limbers the muscles. Warm muscles stretch further, but don't let them trick you into overstretching. I once pulled a muscle while stretching after a long workout. It felt great—the point of "mild discomfort" was nowhere to be found. But the next morning I woke up with a pulled shoulder muscle. Take advantage of your warm muscles and extra flexibility by stretching them only slightly beyond where you normally reach.

DEVELOPMENTAL STRETCHING IS AN EXERCISE IN ITS OWN RIGHT

Developmental stretching, as the name suggests, develops flexibility beyond what it already is. It has only one requirement that differs from performance stretching: you must hold the stretching position for more than 30 seconds. Some exercisers mistake performance stretching for developmental stretching. In fact few exercisers know that there are different techniques to stretching. So they whisk through a stretch in 15 seconds, not pushing their limits or even caring to know what they are. This is performance stretching. If you do it as part of your pre-exercise warm-up, you are using it correctly. If you are trying to increase your flexibility with it, you are wasting your time.

As with cardio exercises, you should do developmental stretches at least three times a week, but when you become flexible enough, you can cut back to once a week, stretching only those muscles that are not exercised in your regular workouts. The muscles exercised in your regular workouts should have their flexibility maintained by the performance stretching part of the warm-up.

I consider developmental stretching to be a form of exercise, and, like any exercise, it should be preceded by a warm-up. The only time you should developmental stretch is when your muscles are thoroughly warmed. Earlier I said that muscles are coldest in the morning and that they warm up as the day continues, but never should you come home in the evening and assume that your muscles are warm enough to developmental stretch. Remember, with developmental stretching you are pushing slightly past your limit. What would happen if you stretched a cold rubber band? It would snap—much more easily than if it were warm. The same thing happens with connective tissue. If you stretch a muscle that's cold, its connective tissue could snap like a cold rubber band.

Give developmental stretching time to show results. No exercise strengthens your muscles or conditions your cardiovascular system overnight. So be patient. It could take one to three months to noticeably increase your flexibility. Considering how long you've neglected your flexibility, that's not much time. (See Figure 6.4 for the ten steps of developmental stretching.)

Figure 6.4   ***DEVELOPMENTAL STRETCHING***

---

1. Wear comfortable clothing allowing easy movement through a full range of motion.

2. Focus on relaxing your body.

3. Breathe in a relaxed, consistent manner as deeply as is comfortable.

4. Slowly and deliberately assume the stretch posture making sure you feel the stretch in the intended location. Stretch only to mild discomfort.

5. Avoid locking joints such as knees. It is unecessary and will save you wear and tear.

6. Avoid arching your back or neck. These maneuvers are only for the very flexible individual doing advanced stretches for specific reasons. If you don't have a reason, don't do it.

7. Maintain the stretch for 30 to 90 seconds.

8. Slowly come out of the stretch.

9. Rest for 10 seconds.

10. Repeat steps 1 through 8 for the same stretch.

If you enjoy stretching, but crave a challenge to energize its passive nature, try PNF (proprioceptive neuromuscular fascilitory) stretching. A difficult technique to master, PNF stretching has two advantages over my six-step method: it is more intense and it gives you quicker results. Rejoice all you impatient people, but also put on your technical thinking caps.

The PNF procedure is built on the principle that the more relaxed a muscle is the better it stretches. As its first step, tense the muscle to be stretched for 10 to 15 seconds. This tires the muscle and helps it to relax. The next step—and this is where it gets technical—requires you to identify muscles in sets of agonist-antagonist classifications based on the anatomical arrangements and the opposing movements that they produce. The antagonist of the quadriceps (front thigh muscle) are the hamstrings (back thigh muscle). When the quadriceps tighten, the hamstrings automatically relax to give it more leeway. Therefore, by purposely tightening the antagonist of the muscle you are stretching, you can relax it more and stretch it farther.

This discussion of PNF stretching isn't meant to give you enough guidance to do it; it's meant to introduce you to, and give you a taste of an advanced stretching technique that you may some day want to try. Obviously, PNF stretching isn't for everyone. What sounds like a good idea to one person may sound like too much trouble to another. If you are in the "too much trouble" group, stick with my simpler but slower six-step method.

GOOD POSTURE IS A RESULT OF BALANCED MUSCULAR FITNESS

A close relative of flexibility is posture. If you are very inflexible, chances are that your posture suffers, though it may also suffer from bad habits and muscle imbalances. Posture is a statement about yourself to the world; it greatly affects the way you look and feel. Yet knowing this, people with poor posture persist in their ways. They refuse to change even when it would add inches to their height or rid them of pain caused by posture-related maladies: an improperly curved spine, slouched shoulders, and an abnormally tilted pelvis. The reason: posture is a very difficult thing to change.

Still, if you do it bit by bit, beginning with the chair you work in and ending with your fitness program, changing your posture is possible. A good chair is the training wheels of your posture, and what it costs or looks like has nothing to do with how well it does this job. Your chair should support you firmly in the small of your back, allowing your spine to maintain its proper curve and your pelvis to be tilted forward so that you sit with your weight off of your tailbone. Its height should allow your thighs to be parallel to the floor when your feet are flat on the ground. This is what your body likes—the position it was made to be in. Give it a chair like this for several months and you will be able to sit with good posture even when you don't have the back support.

A major contributor to poor posture is subtle muscle imbalances. In general, these evolve when your lifestyle concentrates on a narrow scope of activities. Exercisers take this news with disbelief. How could such a good activity create a problem? But activity itself does not ensure that your muscles will develop properly balanced, especially if there are only one or two activities in question. One not-so-subtle example of this is some weight lifters. Built by an unwise weight-lifting program, their huge shoulders hunch forward toward their equally huge chests. Instead, their shoulders should be drawn back by their back muscles, and their lower backs should be supported by their stomach muscles, two muscle groups ignored by their workouts. A balanced strength-training program will naturally improve posture.

Strength training isn't the only kind of exercise that causes muscle imbalances; aerobic exercises also cause them. Go to any race and look at the runners. Many of them will have nice strong legs and for good reason. But look at their upper bodies, so concave and wasted—a muscle imbalance more general than the weight lifters' as it involves the entire upper body, not just some of its muscle groups. What your posture will benefit from, what your body needs, is a balanced exercise program that addresses all major muscle groups rather than a select few.

Of course, a balanced fitness program would not be complete without flexibility. Good flexibility through stretching helps your posture by releasing your body to assume its natural alignment, and it's a release, that for many people, can't happen too soon. Living with poor posture is like living in prison. Yet people grow used to this kind of life; they find it comfortable. They don't realize that many of their aches and pains are an outgrowth of it.

Poor posture does more than pain the body; it pains the mind. A slumped shoulder, somewhat hunched back look seems to say that you are bearing the worries of the world on your shoulders—and crumbling beneath them. Day after day your body performs a pantomime that says, "I can't cope. I can't handle it." And everybody listens—your family, your friends, your boss, your coworkers, and worst of all your own mind. When your body tells your brain it's overwhelmed, your brain believes it. But standing tall, head up, shoulders back, you give your brain the opposite message and from it comes a surge of confidence.

Never underestimate the power of the mind. Several years ago a friend injured his back while putting a heavy bag in an overhead bin on an airplane. Two weeks of anti-inflammatory medication, some hot packs, and massages set his back right; but it was his observation, not his recovery, that was illustrative. If he walked without any bounce, from side to side, he had no pain. This together with the knowledge that his back was getting better and the general state of his life—a successful career and a thriving family—were all reasons for him to be happy. Why, then, did he feel so depressed? Because he was *acting* depressed. His posture and his movements were the same as those of severely depressed people, though with them it works the other way around; their posture and movements are imposed on them by their depressed minds. Between the mind and body there is a two-way street.

Flexibility is the easiest solution to the everyday muscular and skeletal problems that sap your psychic energy. By improving it through stretching, you brighten your mood and sharpen your mind. Use the knowledge you now have to design a balanced exercise program that includes flexibility. Build it into your goals. Include it in your warm-ups. Shape it into a workout. Let it recapture your youth and keep you fresh and alert.

• CHAPTER 7 •

EXERCISING OPTIONS

"How can I exercise? I'm too busy rolling out a new product or flying somewhere like Seattle, where it's always raining, or Minnesota, where it gets 20 below zero," said Pete, looking as haggard as he sounded. "Besides," he continued, "my knee is acting up again, so I might as well give it a rest. All I can do is try to make up for it later." Pete, the vice president of sales for his company, is struggling to fit a running program into his life, but "something" always seems to interfere. There are many reasons to skip exercising, and some of them are valid. But most are excuses.

More than ever, today's executives face the temptation to skip exercise; they must contend with four major roadblocks—time, injury, travel, and weather—which together are enough to discourage even the most avid exerciser. Yet there are ways to overcome all of them.

In Chapter 3, "Creating Time for Fitness," I show you how to overcome the time crunch. In Chapter 10, "Preventing Injuries," I study the injury nemesis so devastating to beginners and longtime exercisers alike, that some studies rank it the number one reason people give up exercise. With injuries an ounce of prevention is worth a pound of cure. But the primary focus of this chapter,

111

"Exercising Options," is on the weather and travel roadblocks—after all, where else is a busy executive more likely to find a roadblock than on the road?

CROSS-TRAINING GRANTS YOU OPTIONS TO EXERCISE

What you need to overcome these obstacles are options—not the kind that reward you financially—but options that allow you to pursue exercise in spite of everyday life. One option granter is cross-training. The idea of cross-training is, to many new exercisers, intimidating. They conjure up images of a superfit triathlete, swimming, biking, running and generally performing like an exerciser extraordinaire. But strictly speaking, cross-training means consistently doing more than one kind of exercise, and many veteran exercisers do it to maintain peak interest in their primary exercise while avoiding overuse injuries.

Cross-training gives you another benefit; it injects flexibility into your program. Say, for example, that you cross-country ski (on a simulator) for aerobic exercise and discover on a business trip that the hotel's fitness room has only exercycles, a treadmill, and a multistation weight-lifting machine. Do you throw up your hands and skip the workout? Or do you get on an exercycle, which you never use, and desperately peddle up a sweat? The answer to both is no. Exercises are muscle specific. Put untrained muscles to the task of providing vigorous workouts, and you risk an injury or at the very least a stiff, painful awakening the next morning. Don't approach an exercise you never do with random abandon. Plan to do another exercise by cross-training with it first. This will not only acclimate your muscles to the exercise; it will also give your mind a chance to learn the workout intensity that induces a heart-healthy pulse rate. An experienced runner knows how fast he has to run to reach a certain percent of his pulse limit. Put that runner on a bike and he'll have no idea what percent he's reached; he'll think he's exercising on one level while his heart is on another. Well conditioned, his heart can tolerate cycling far better than a nonexerciser's heart. But it gets a confusing message from his leg muscles. Some of those muscles are untrained and can't use oxygen as efficiently peddling a bike. What would have been enough oxygen for running is not enough oxygen for cycling, and the heart is told to beat faster. Being trained for one exercise does not mean you are trained specifically enough for another.

Think, too, of how you would feel if you had to settle for an alien workout. It would be impossible to look forward to, and you'd feel aggravated and bored. But when you're familiar with an exercise, your mind anticipates doing it with as much joy as it would doing your primary exercise. It's a law of nature.

Because the condition of your cardiovascular system is so important, make your first cross-training exercise an aerobic one. Trauma medicine illustrates this point perfectly. For example, if a patient cannot breathe, repairing a wound in the arm will do little to save his life. Always establish an airway first; this is what life depends on. The same is true with fitness. First address the heart of the matter. Then go for the total package by striving for muscular strength, endurance, and flexibility. Taken in that order, your fitness program expands effortlessly. Once a person is committed to cardio fitness, having established a habit that encourages him to get a heart-healthy workout by "hook or by crook," he is far more likely to move into other areas of fitness, like muscular strength, for the challenge and achievement of it.

Figure 7.1 suggests cross-training matches for a variety of primary exercises. But ultimately the choice is yours. What you choose should be the exercises that keep you from getting bored and give you the most flexibility. Then, as an executive trained for several exercises, you'll no longer see roadblocks as formidable detours in your exercise program; you'll just jump right over them.

RUNNING ON-THE-ROAD

Running is the most popular aerobic exercise in the United States. One of the reasons is its convenience; it can be done practically anywhere. For travelers such portability is a blessing—just pack your running shoes and seasonal running clothes and race off to a workout as enjoyable as it is effective at conditioning the heart.

Whether running is a primary or cross-training exercise, you will encounter some differences doing it on-the-road, such as the roads themselves. If you're not familiar with the neighborhood, note

---

Figure 7.1   ***CROSS-TRAINING COMBINATIONS***

Aerobic-Anaerobic: for balance

Running	Upper body weight lifting
Cycling	Upper body weight lifting
Cross-country skiing *	Upper body weight lifting
Stairclimbing	Upper body weight lifting
Rowing	Lower body weight lifting
Swimming	Lower body weight lifting

* Assumes you don't use the poling attachment

Aerobic-Aerobic: to supplement primary exercise

Running	Racewalking, stairclimbing (instead of speedwork), aerobics
Cycling	Cross-country skiing, stairclimbing
Cross-country skiing	Cycling, stairclimbing
Stairclimbing	Cycling, running, aerobics

Aerobic-Aerobic: to complement primary exercise

Running	Cross-country skiing, cycling, rowing, swimming
Cycling	Running, rowing, swimming, aerobics
Cross-country skiing	Running, rowing, swimming, aerobics
Stairclimbing	Rowing, racewalking, swimming
Rowing	Cycling, running, cross-country skiing, stairclimbing, swimming, aerobics
Aerobics	Cycling, cross-country skiing, rowing, swimming

possible running routes as you approach the hotel, but beware of the temptation to explore—it can turn a short run into a long search for home. Always ask the natives where it's safe and easy to run. Such indigenous input can be a life-saver. Take New York's Central Park, for example. At 7:00 A.M. it's safe; after dark avoid it unless you're running with a squad of heavily armed commandos. Any New Yorker will tell you that.

A run can give you more than exercise. Use it to scout the territory and get your bearings. Note stores, restaurants, client offices, their suppliers, and competitors. You'll be surprised how many times you'll notice something that will be useful later, either to yourself or in conversations with others.

Travel schedules may force you to depart from your normal running time. In a city of any size, outdoor running is usually safer when done in the early morning, before rush hour hits and pollution settles in. Pollution from cars won't dissipate until traffic thins out again late at night. Even tree-lined suburban areas sequester pollution. If you have a choice, run in open areas that are less landscaped; they tend to hold less pollution.

What to pack for an activity is always an important issue when you travel, and if you run outdoors, the weather will always dictate it. In warm weather all you need is a pair of well-broken-in running shoes (a hotel is no place to be doctoring blisters), socks, shorts, and a T-shirt. Cold weather is a little more complicated. Exactly how cold is it? Wind and rain lower the perceived temperature to your body. But a rain suit, a sweat suit, a hat, and a pair of gloves are light and take up little space. Even more compact is the plastic laundry bag found in most hotel closets. Use it as a handy divider to pack your soiled running clothes in for the trip home.

The convenience of running on-the-road also holds for a similar exercise, racewalking. Racewalking's advantage over running is that it is a relatively low-impact exercise that can be performed by people with arthritic problems of the lower back, hips, legs, and feet. By walking regularly, some people with arthritic knees have improved their joints' flexibility and decreased their pain. And race-walking involves less impact than regular walking, yet gives your heart a more vigorous workout. That makes it one of the gentle heroes of the exercise brigade.

CHECKING OUT FITNESS FACILITIES

But you can't always count on running or racewalking the roads of the city you visit—the weather may veto it, or your schedule may crowd it out of safe times. In these cases look for an indoor option.

Hotel Fitness Centers

Before you make reservations at a hotel, ask about its fitness facility. When does it open? A survey in New York, Chicago, and Los Angeles showed that most hotels open their fitness centers between 6:00 and 6:45 A.M., and close them between 9:00 (most common) and 11:00 P.M.—reasonable hours for both early bird and nocturnal exercisers.

The quality of the fitness center is another question. To know that a hotel has a fitness center open at decent times isn't enough; the kind of equipment also counts. Some fitness centers may have an impressive array of aerobic equipment, from treadmills and stair-climbers to rowers and exercycles, complemented by strength-building equipment like free weights, multistation weight machines, or single-station circuit machines. Other fitness centers may be more limited or even off premises.

Hotels without fitness centers often make arrangements with outside fitness clubs to accept their guests. Sometimes free, sometimes for a small fee, the arrangement may at first seem inconvenient, but on closer examination it is often a blessing. Most independent health clubs have a larger and newer array of equipment. It's their business and your advantage.

In San Antonio I stayed at a hotel that had such an arrangement. The fitness club was a 4-minute walk away and charged $5 per guest visit. The hotel charged as little as $50 a night. That should tell you that you don't have to stay at a luxury hotel to have access to a fitness center. In fact, the difference in price between a hotel with a fitness room and one without a fitness room will not be a factor in deciding where you stay.

You can find a hotel with a fitness center; the question is how to find a hotel with a quality one? Is the equipment high quality and well kept, or is it broken down or worn out? Is there enough equipment, or do you often have to wait? Is the place clean? Unfortunately you won't get answers to these questions over the phone; you can only find out by going there. Most business travelers visit the same city time after time. Therefore it will pay to keep track of your accommodations by noting the quality of a hotel's facilities on 3″ by 5″ cards or on your personal computer (see Figure 7.2). Some will be winners; some will be losers. While you're compiling your list, you will be in an experimental phase, and your fitness program will not always benefit. Be patient. The time spent finding good hotel fitness centers is an investment in your future.

Figure 7.2   SAMPLE 3" x 5" CARD FOR FITNESS CENTERS

Name of Hotel:

Fitness Facility:	No	Yes	Hours

Equipment:

	Aerobic:	(e.g., Treadmill, exercycle, stairclimber, rower)
	Anaerobic:	(e.g., Single-station or multistation weight machine, free weights)

Comments:	(e.g., Clean, good condition, enough equipment)

Commercial Gyms

After having completed your list, you might find that certain cities have "losers" only. Before settling for a second-rate workout, consider another option: a commercial gym. Commercial gyms are located in most cities, and even though different gyms will have different rules, it's quite likely you'll be able to find a suitable arrangement within a reasonable distance from your hotel. In fact, first find a gym; then make reservations at a hotel near it.

As an example of what you can find, Gold's Gym has many well-equipped facilities throughout the country. Most Gold Gyms (it may vary from gym to gym) offer one free visit to anyone who walks in. After that a nonmember must pay $10 for each visit. Given the quality of the equipment, that's quite reasonable. Membership, however, does have its privileges, A Gold's Gym member who is over 50 miles from his or her home gym can use an out-of-town gym for up to two weeks at no charge. Similar arrangements are bound to be available with other commercial establishments. The point is that you can find an excellent gym on the road regardless of what your hotel offers.

Start by asking any gyms in your hometown for a copy of their rules and a list of out-of-town locations. If you don't find any in the city you are planning to visit, go through the Yellow Pages at that destination. Unless your hotel is in the middle of a Kansas wheat field, you should find a gym nearby.

Using Out-of-Town Facilities

Whether the gym you use is a hotel spa or an outside fitness club, it's the exercise you do at it that counts. What exercise will that be? If you're a runner, you might choose your primary exercise by using the treadmill. Or you might cross-train, peddling on an exercycle, rowing on a rower, gliding on a cross-country ski machine, or stepping up a stairclimber. As long as you are properly trained, anything goes.

That includes weight lifting. If your job regularly takes you out of town one or two days a week, a well-equipped gym may be exactly what you need to cross-train anaerobically. Concentrate on the areas of the body missed by your aerobic workout. For runners, cyclers, and stairclimbers, that would be your entire upper body. For rowers and cross-country skiers, it would be certain muscles of the arms, chest, and shoulders. You don't have to balance your muscles by power lifting with very heavy weights. If you row and cross-country ski, power lifting would make the weaker muscles too strong for the aerobically exercised ones, creating a muscle imbalance just the opposite of the one you are trying to correct. As for runners and other exercisers whose entire upper bodies are weak, power lifting is still unnecessary. Endurance weight lifting—the low-weight, high-rep kind—is enough.

Assuming that you can lift weights once a week at home, you need only to lift them one more time each week to continue your muscular growth. Even with a heavy travel schedule, you can build strength. Would you lose any strength if your travels took you to a remote location where there was no gym or where your schedule left no time to use one? The answer is no. One workout a week is enough to maintain the strength you already have. When your schedule lightens, you can continue to build.

CLEVER USE OF HOTEL FACILITIES

Some exercise opportunities won't be as obvious as finding a convenient gym, but if you keep an alert eye on your surroundings you may discover some options.

Up the Down Escalator

Take escalators, for example. Many hotels in major cities have them in the main lobby, between the ground and first or second floors. They are there to save your energy; use them, instead, to expend it. Early in the morning when traffic is light, walk up the down escalator for a stairclimbing workout comparable to what you could get on a stairclimbing machine. Either way you get nowhere, but your cardiovascular system will end up in good enough condition to get you anywhere.

If you can't use an escalator, try the stairs. This requires, first, that you check at the desk to make sure they are safe and, second (assuming that they *are* safe), that you somehow sustain the workout for 20 minutes. If the hotel has many floors, your strategy is simple: walk up for 20 minutes. If the hotel doesn't have enough floors for this, guard your knees. Few activities are more stressful to the knees than walking or running downstairs, and no workout, heart healthy or not, should include it. Still, this kind of stairclimbing demands that what goes up must also come down. One option is to take the elevator, running in place to keep your heart rate up while waiting for it to come and while on it.

Clearly this strategy won't work if the elevator is crowded or you have to use it several times. Another option is to use what I call the stair stretching technique. On your way up, take two steps up and one step down, always facing up the staircase. Stepping down one step at a time is easier on the knees than descending a flight at a time; it decreases the downward momentum, which lessens the impact. A backward step down also requires more energy, develops the renowned knee-supporting quadriceps, and stresses the knee less. But follow the procedure exactly as outlined. If you go up one step or three steps and then down one, you'll always be stepping down with the same leg. That concentrates the burden on one leg. You want it shared by both.

Swim-Running

Stairclimbing, however, isn't for everyone, especially if escalators bore you and stairwells give you the creeps. What is a harried traveler to do then, relax by the pool? Well, almost. Head for the pool, yes. Relax, no. Not that you should jump in for a long swim. As I pointed out in Chapter 4, swimming requires easy access to a pool year round, and most people don't have that. But nowadays pools are being used for another exercise, swim-running. An outgrowth of rehabilitating injuries, swim-running has two advantages: it is non-impact, making it easier on the joints and tendons, and it gives your upper body a respectable workout because of the water's resistance to your arms as they pump.

Though swim-running is a vigorous exercise that's easy on the body, your heart rate won't tell you how vigorous until you adjust it. The cooling effect of water lowers the heart rate as much as 25 percent of what it would be for the same work intensity in air. At the same time the heaviness of water lulls you into running at a lower speed. With these two factors working together, your heart rate may stay so low that you wonder why you are bothering to do this exercise at all. But these are really illusions. You *are* exercising. You *are* accomplishing something. So don't become unnerved. Just concentrate on maintaining your speed and shoot for a heart rate that's 20 percent lower than your normal exercise rate.

Most runners won't have the opportunity to swim-run at home. Hotel pools will be your only training sites. Hence you should acclimate your body to it slowly by cutting your initial workout times in half and taking 1-minute breaks after each 5-minute bout of exercise. This gentle introduction also allows you to practice the technique so you have it down by the time you are ready to extend your workout. "But," you may ask, "if I already run, why do I need to practice?"

The technique of swim-running differs from that of land running. Instead of leaning slightly forward, as in the conventional running posture, your body should remain straight with your feet pointed downward throughout your stride. Your arm motion is more restricted than regular running. Keeping your arms bent at an 80-degree angle, you swing your elbows in a 45- to 50-degree arc from the front of your chest to slightly past your back, while your hands remain open with palms facing down so they can slice through the water.

To swim-run, you should be in deep enough water to prevent your feet from touching the bottom. That means you need a flotation vest. There are many on the market. What you want is the one that packs most easily. Another piece of gear you'll need is a tether, which you can buy or make out of a nylon rope and any flexible tubing, like a bicycle wheel's inner tube. By tying the flexible end around yourself just below the chest, or around the waist if the flotation vest is in the way, and the other end to something on the side of the pool, you anchor yourself to one spot. It is unlikely you will be the only one in the hotel pool. But nobody should begrudge your "running" in one spot, off to the side.

If swim-running doesn't at first sound like a good exercise option, then, of course, pursue one that does. But don't dismiss swim-running completely; file it in the back of your mind. It could become a valuable option if you ever get injured.

HANG THE "DO NOT DISTURB" SIGN ON YOUR DOORKNOB

One hotel "facility" that's always available to you is your room. In your room you can exercise your heart so effectively, it won't matter if there isn't a fitness center for miles.

Slideboarding

One fairly new exercise easily done in your room is slideboarding. By sliding laterally from one side of a mat to the other, using a form similar to a speedskater's, you can get a workout as rigorous as cross-country skiing or running. All you need is a slideboard—a five-foot mat with bumpers on each edge—and low-friction "booties" or shoe covers that act as skates.

What makes this such a good travel option is its portability. The slideboard rolls up. The booties fold. And the music tape you could carry in your coat pocket. I suggest you take music along, because there is a tendency to slow down without a guiding tempo. As a relatively low-impact exercise, slideboarding should stand out as a pearl among travel options. Done in the privacy of your room, at your convenience, it can be squeezed into the tightest schedule.

Aerobic Dance

A popular exercise you can do in your room is aerobic dance, but doing it on-the-road does require some preparation. First select a video routine that you enjoy, and practice it as part of your home workout to familiarize yourself with the moves and cues. Then record the video's audio portion. VCRs in hotel rooms are quite rare—they would compete with the in-room movies. An audio tape, with the help of your memory, will give you the vocal cues you need.

Of course, many people may think it's easier to just tune into a morning exercise program since most areas of the country have them. Easier, yes—safer no. From a TV routine, you really don't know what to expect. The ones I watched were very demanding, like preparatory courses for Marine boot camp, and you would have to be superbly fit to get through them. The best outcome of following such a program is that you are *only* sore the next day. In aerobic dance you can never play it too safe. Bring your own audio tape.

Stretching

Complete your on-the-road fitness program with performance stretching exercises. Done before or after you work out, they will keep you limber. Done before bed, they can relax you to sleep. Or you might want to graduate from performance stretching to developmental stretching—another perfect in-room exercise—and improve the flexibility of your entire body.

With so many options to exercise when you travel, no circumstance can prevent you from exercising—if you really want to. That is the stickler: you must want to. But wanting to exercise when you are traveling and tired and perhaps out of sorts from bouncing between time zones isn't always the easiest thing to do. What you need is a goal and a habit. If you commit yourself to the goal, if you plan out how to do it, if you do what you planned, something unexpected will happen: you'll find yourself looking forward to exercising on-the-road. Traveling never felt so good. (See Figure 7.3 for a review of all these exercise options.)

Figure 7.3   **ON-THE-ROAD EXERCISE OPTIONS**

Running	Highly portable exercise you can do almost anywhere. Excellent for getting your bearings in new cities. Pick safe courses and low traffic times to run.
Fitness Center	Becoming more prevalent in hotels with accommodating hours. If unable to find a hotel with suitable facilities seek out nearby commercial gyms. Use cross-training workouts such as exercycle, stairclimbing, rowing, or weight lifting. Become acclimated to specific exercise at home before doing it on the road.
Stairclimbing	Walking up the down escalator (traffic and facilities permitting) or up the hotel staircase (sufficient number of flights and safe) provides an excellent workout if other options are not available.
Swim-Running	Increasing in popularity as an excellent exercise if you're injured or want to avoid injuries. Pack a flotation vest and tether to run in place in the deep-water end of the hotel pool. Take it easy as a beginner while learning the proper technique.
Slideboarding	Very convenient to pack a slideboard and special "booties" or shoe covers and exercise in your room quietly and privately. Take along a music tape or CD to help you keep your tempo.
Aerobics	Exercise in the privacy of your hotel room but prepare in advance by learning your routine at home and bringing your own audio tape. A routine you find on your hotel TV may be too challenging unless you're an advanced aerobic dancer.
Stretching	Whether performance or developmental stretching, this perfectly portable activity can be done almost anywhere without requiring a long uninterrupted period of exercise time.

NEITHER RAIN, NOR SLEET, NOR SNOW...

Using weather as an excuse to skip exercise is about as common as using travel. I have noticed that outdoor exercisers tend to talk more about the weather than two strangers on an elevator—it's raining, it's snowing, it's too cold, it's too hot and humid. True, there are some weather conditions where you need to seek shelter and protection, not exercise and enjoyment, but those conditions tend to be rare: hurricanes, lightning, tornadoes, blizzards, and ice storms. Yet even during these furies of nature you can usually exercise indoors, either with the machine version of your primary workout or with a cross-training routine.

Many people use a double standard on weather: what's OK for some activities is not good for exercise. Consider the throngs of people who sit in the cold rain on Saturdays and Sundays each fall, soaking in the football contests of their choosing. Or how about all the glowing vacationers I share the freezing slopes with in Aspen, Colorado, skiing in the powdery, high-altitude snow? If all these fun-loving people can get out in "bad" weather, why can't they exercise in it? The answer is they can. It's a matter of attitude, of wanting to exercise as in wanting to cheer at a football game or ski at a winter resort.

Rainy Days

It's also a matter of what to wear. Much of the problem of exercising in bad weather can be solved by dressing properly. In rain, a hood, a billed hat, or a full-rimmed hat will keep your head dry and your eyes clear. A rainsuit made of Gore-Tex™, Microfine®, or Sympatex®, breathable yet water-impermeable fabrics, keeps the rest of your body dry. Except for the feet.

Finding the right footwear is the trickiest part of dressing for the rain; most running shoes—and both runners and walkers should wear them—are not rainproof. But some brands do stay drier than others. While one pair of shoes will seemingly suck the fog out of the air and concentrate it on your toes, another pair will keep your feet dry in a light rain. Experiment with the different shoe designs and materials until you find a pair that keeps your feet relatively dry.

Still, it shouldn't be a tragedy if your feet get wet; just plan your workout accordingly. Don't run too fast or stay out too long, especially if you have a problem with your toes rubbing together. Let logic govern when you exercise in the rain. If you're dressed properly, it can be a comfortable—even cozy—experience.

Bikers, too, must deal with rain, though here the paramount issue is safety. A biker's speed makes wind a factor. Combined with wind, rain greatly reduces visibility, both frontal and peripheral. Meanwhile your stopping distance also lengthens. All of which is not to say that you shouldn't ride in the rain, but that you should dress properly and practice safety.

Searing Summers

Sun, heat, and humidity are potential hazards, and they should be treated that way (see Figure 7.4). When you exercise, your body increases its heat production 10- to 20-fold. As its inner temperature rises it sweats, covering the skin with fluid that cools the body by evaporating. In warm weather you sweat more for more cooling evaporation. It's as if your body runs its own biological air conditioner, a design so ingenious that it self-adjusts for the weather. Only nature could have designed this—but it's not foolproof. It won't work well if you don't drink enough because fluids ingested are the primary source of sweat, or if the humidity is too high, because evaporation won't take place. I compare it to running a car without oil; eventually, the engine will overheat and seize.

Still, hot weather is a fact of life for many of you, and if you want to overcome the roadblock of exercising outdoors, take the following steps.

1. Acclimatize your body with at least two weeks of less intense exercise under warm, humid conditions.

2. Drink plenty of fluids: 12 to 16 ounces about a half hour before exercise and 3 to 6 ounces every 15 minutes to 30 minutes thereafter. Don't drink soda or fruit juices—the sugar content is too high and will interfere with absorption. If you crave sweet flavor, drink a sugarless beverage. As for "sports drinks," they have no advantage over plain water at keeping you cool.

3. Exercise in the earliest part of the day. It is the coolest time. The sun's rays are weaker and therefore less damaging to the skin.

4. Wear loose, light-colored clothing made of a cotton-polyester blend. In sunlight men should never exercise bare-chested and women should not wear those bra-like sports tops. Besides absorbing more radiant heat than a light colored shirt, bare skin absorbs the sun's UV rays, which can cause skin cancer. Also protect your head by wearing a white-billed cap to reflect sun.

Harsh Winters

At the opposite end of the thermometer is the problem of exercising in the cold (see Figure 7.4). Usually cold weather isn't as dangerous as hot weather. It's a question of dressing up. The secret is to dress in layers, with the layer closest to your body made of a fabric that wicks sweat from the skin and passes it on to the next layer, allowing your skin to remain fairly dry. Sporting goods stores and catalogs sell this fabric under the generic name polypropylene. Over polypropylene you place another layer that absorbs the sweat and insulates. Wool, cotton, synthetic fibers like acrylic and polyester or blends of each perform both duties well, and as the temperature drops, these are the fabrics you add more layers of because they trap air between them and trapped air acts as insulation.

Figure 7.4	EXERCISING IN EXTREME TEMPERATURES
Heat	Wear loose, light-colored clothing and a billed hat. Drink 12–16 ounces of fluid one-half hour before exercise and 3–6 ounces every 15 to 30 minutes thereafter. Reduce intensity and duration of workout.
Cold	Dress in layers of clothing: polypropylene next to the skin, then cotton or cotton blend in one or more layers, topped with windproof shell. Cover your head including nose, mouth, and ears. Wear double layer of gloves and socks. Reduce intensity and duration of workout.

The last, or outer layer, should be a protective shell that breaks the wind. For this you can use the jacket of your rainsuit or any light shell that is windproof. Shells come in two basic styles: pull-over and zipper-down. Judging by what I see for sale, I would think that the pull-over style is more popular. If it is, I don't know why. A shell with a full-length zipper is more versatile and convenient because it allows you to keep part of the layer on while letting cool air through the front if it gets too warm. Overheat in the pull-over style and you have to remove the entire layer, which may be too much.

The legs aren't as sensitive as the upper body is to cold. But in extreme cold, they too will need pants of the same shell material to block the wind from chilling them.

That takes care of your arms, legs, and torso. Even more important to keep warm are your head, hands, and feet. If it's not too cold, a light-weight toboggan-style hat, an inexpensive pair of cotton garden gloves, and thick socks may be all you need. But in harsh subfreezing temperatures the hands and feet are hard to keep warm, and unless properly protected quite vulnerable to frostbite. Apply the layering system here too. Cover your hands with a first layer of thin silk gloves. Over them wear thick wool mittens, sealed off from the cold by an outer layer of rain and windproof shell. Use a similar layering system on the feet. Cover a thin pair of inner socks with a thick pair of outer socks. But none of this will keep your hands or feet warm if the rest of your upper body is cold. A chill to your body will cause your brain to signal for the withdrawal of blood from the extremities, and no matter how many layers your hands and feet have on them, they will feel cold.

The head has the opposite problem. With a rich blood supply unaffected by the rest of the body's warmth, it tends to feel warm in cold weather. Many people misinterpret this. They think, "If my head feels warm, everything is OK." Everything isn't OK. An uncovered head can lead to massive loss of body heat. Again and again, I see skiers make this mistake as they schuss down the slopes without hats. They are colder than they look. Always wear one, if not two, layers on your head and ears, and if the weather is cold enough, add a layer of protection to the face, particularly the nose and mouth. I wear a ski face mask. It protects my skin from freezing and helps warm the air as I breathe it in.

Snow is yet another weather condition you must deal with. Walking or running in a winter wonderland may be beautiful, but it also requires decent footing—a reasonably clear path free of ice and traffic. If you don't have this, exercise another option. That goes for cycling too. I learned this lesson the hard way when the rear end of my bike spun out without warning. Only an inch of snow was on the ground, yet I wondered how I could make it home safely. I still cycle when it snows, but indoors on my exercycle.

As you exercise, your body generates great amounts of heat, which makes the air temperature feel warmer than it really is. Then there are many weather combinations that affect how cold it feels— sun, wind, humidity all conspire with the temperature to create the cold you must dress for. This makes it difficult to know how to dress. Let experience be your guide. But if you are ever unsure of what to wear, remember this golden rule of cold weather dressing: it is better to overdress than to underdress.

High Altitude

Cold weather brings to mind a favorite activity of executives from all over the United States—skiing. Picture the executive from New Jersey on a recreational ski vacation. He travels to the Rockies for the ultimate in powder skiing, fully intending to ski down every trail of the mountain in one day. But something happens once he gets there: his Olympian goals are squashed by a lack of energy. He wonders if he's coming down with something. What the skier is feeling is the effect of altitude. At higher altitudes, the air contains less oxygen. Not only does this decrease your capacity to exercise— a specific exercise intensity at sea level is harder to perform at 2,000 feet—it can make you very ill. Headaches, nausea, insomnia, restlessness, blurry vision, palpitations, and poor appetite are all symptoms of an illness called Acute Mountain Sickness (AMS). Probably you won't suffer from all these symptoms. Any symptoms you do have, however, will be worsened by exercise.

AMS is not a permanent response to altitude; eventually the body adapts and the symptoms disappear. But "eventually" could mean as long as a month, and most visitors to higher altitudes don't have that much time. Therefore, to feel your best and be able to exercise without becoming ill, eat more carbohydrates and much less protein. Drink plenty of fluids—at least 16 cups a day, excluding alcohol. Alcohol is a diuretic—just the opposite of what you need—and at high altitudes it affects your brain even more. You don't need that either. Finally, cut back on the intensity and duration of your workout.

That last piece of advice, cutting back on your exercise, is an option you should practice in all nonroutine circumstances. Whether you're running in a strange city, lifting weights on a new machine in a hotel gym, or exercising in the harsh elements of nature, a cautious approach is the option to exercise.

Like Pete, the sales VP at the beginning of this chapter, most executives are the focal point of a tug-of-war waged by external demands. On one end is their careers, consuming their mental and physical energy, sending them all over the United States and perhaps the world and monopolizing their time. On the other end is their personal lives, their families, their friends, their leisure activities—their health. And let's not forget Mother Nature with her tricky weather, at times fiendishly tugging on both ends. As an executive you are self-motivated to do what's right for your career. What's right for your career is exercise. It's also right for every other part of your life. In the past, the tug-of-war built roadblocks to exercise so high and so wide that they may have seemed insurmountable; you had neither the means nor the opportunity to hurdle them. Now you have both in the form of options. Your job is to make sure you exercise those options so you can proceed toward your vision of a longer, healthier, more productive life.

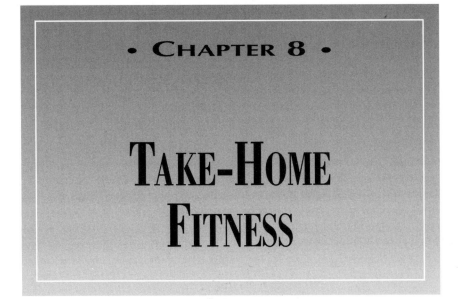

· CHAPTER 8 ·

TAKE-HOME
FITNESS

A decade ago home gyms were primarily limited to private training centers of professional athletes, who used them to sharpen their competitive edge. Today they are an affordable convenience used to save time. Thanks to consumer demand, the exercise industry, which once made equipment for fitness clubs or commercial gyms only, now turns out noncommercial versions of their equipment for home use. And business has been booming. For several years, the annual sale of home fitness products has topped over $2 billion. This recent demand is rooted in the realization fitness isn't just a way to look good; it's a way to improve your productivity and preserve your health.

But the evolution of exercise from a pastime of health nuts to a priority in life is incomplete and will remain so until exercise is as important as eating and sleeping. Take-home meals are popular because of their convenience. Now it's time for exercise to become just as popular—and important—because of the convenience of home equipment.

THE CONVENIENCE OF TAKING FITNESS HOME

Convenience means saving time by not driving out of your way to go to a fitness club, and not waiting in line for the machine of your choice, a common occurrence during peak hours. Convenience means exercising any time you want to. At home you can create time by waking up at 5:00 A.M. for a 5:15 A.M. workout; fitness clubs usually won't open before 6:00 A.M. Convenience means being able to have an impromptu workout; 30 minutes suddenly becomes free and your "fitness club" is a few steps away.

Always at the core of convenience is the element of time saved. Home equipment saves even more of it by giving you the option of EXTRAcising. As discussed in Chapter 3, EXTRAcising means doing something else while you exercise such as watching the news, listening to music or educational tapes, baby-sitting, and many other activities you simply couldn't do at a fitness club.

In time value alone home equipment is worth the investment, and the savings run deeper. Consider the total cost of you and your family belonging to a fitness club. Consider too the kind of equipment you want to work out on; at a fitness club you must use what they choose. When you buy it, you can choose exactly what you want—the treadmill with the lowest-impact surface or the stair-climber with the upper body exercise option.

At home you can dress as you please. Exercising at the club or even outdoors requires another level of dress. Unsuitable are those ragged, old clothes that are so comfortable. I always joke that some of the outfits I wear, I wouldn't be seen in moving the sprinkler. Still, those "old favorites" are my most comfortable ones, and they require very little care. Save your spiffy outfits for entertaining an exercise-minded business guest or client; a private exercise session followed by a "working" dinner would be well appreciated by an out-of-towner whose travel interferes with his fitness program.

Perhaps you're a runner or cyclist who can just open the front door and start pumping your legs. That's convenience too. But many of us are not so fortunate. Living where the traffic's too heavy, the hills too steep, or the roads too few, we are literally forced to stay indoors. And even those fortunate few who do live in the perfect neighborhood have to contend with workout-busters like ice, heat and humidity, or lightning. Don't expect Mother Nature to cooperate with your schedule. Put a treadmill or exercycle under your roof for bad weather. Any runner or cyclist who has the option of doing his workouts indoors will tell you how good it feels to not worry about the weather, or to cross-train with a different exercise indoors, making himself less vulnerable to injuries. That's convenience.

Beyond the time and money saved, home equipment offers another perk, this one greater than the other two together: adherence. A home gym allows exercise to fit more easily into your life—to become, in the long run, a priority so important that you wouldn't want to give it up for any reason. This is adherence. A phenomenon clearly defined by scientific research, it is easy to spot in exercisers—they simply hate to miss a workout. That home equipment increases the probability of adherence has also been proven by research, but it's easy enough to prove yourself. Just ask any exerciser what his home equipment means to him. I have a friend I used to call a fair weather runner. In nice weather running was his "passion," but if it so much as drizzled he would call off his workout and pursue other "more important" activities. A treadmill in his home changed all that. Now he races out the door in heavy rain—"it's only water"—to train for races.

How to Select the Right Exercise Equipment for You

Some people, however, defy the adherence rule by letting their exercise equipment lay fallow in their homes. The reason is that they didn't buy the right equipment. When you shop for home equipment, it's easy to become overwhelmed by all the factors to consider—size, price, quality, repair options, as well as the specific features each machine offers. There seems to be as many different machines as there are exercisers, and I have no intention of giving you detailed evaluations of the latest models or prices from different stores or manufacturers. This isn't a monthly consumer magazine. What I will do is steer you in the right direction. To help you decide what to buy, I condensed the many factors involved into three categories: purpose, value, and features. The first two categories are general and apply to all exercise equipment. The third, features, is specific to the particular piece of equipment.

Matching Equipment with Its Purpose

Your attitude toward the equipment you buy will decide whether you use it or not. Many people approach this purchase with an idea of what they *should* buy. It's a common mistake—one that I made. Ten years ago an orthopedic surgeon suggested that I rehabilitate my knees by cycling. At first I didn't think that an exercycle was necessary; outdoor riding was an activity I had always enjoyed as a child, and I committed myself to doing it year round. But a few cases of frostbitten toes and a harrowing ride in the snow convinced me that I shouldn't bike outdoors in winter. Into the house came my first piece of exercise equipment, an exercycle. I *should* have used it. Unfortunately my heart—and my mind—wasn't into the indoor version of cycling, and as the exercycle collected dust in my basement, my swollen knees continued to pain me. Then I learned about the NordicTrack® cross-country ski machine. Into the house came my second piece of equipment—but this time I used it. While its nonpounding motion coddled my knees, I got a gritty workout that made me feel accomplished, and I found myself repeatedly extending my workouts. I also found myself finishing a workout with a 20- or 30-minute ride on the newly dusted exercycle. It, too, became a well-used piece of equipment, but only after I was captured by my favorite machine. The moral of this story: buy what you *want,* not what you think you should. If you enjoy running, buy a treadmill. Don't buy an exercycle because it costs less; you'll just be discounting your own fitness. Buy equipment for an exercise you don't enjoy indoors or at all, and you'll end up watching TV.

Before you buy any equipment ask yourself: "What is its purpose? Will it be the mainstay of my fitness program or a supplement for cross-training? Will I move all my exercise indoors come winter, or will I continue to train outdoors, with occasional stints indoors during bad weather?" Your answers will tell you how much you intend to use the equipment. Your next step is to buy a piece suitable for that level of use. For a primary exercise you'll need a durable piece of equipment because it will be used more, and with durability usually comes more bulk, more weight, and a higher price.

Some beginners may be unsure about which exercise will ultimately be their primary one. How can you choose equipment when you don't know what you'll need? I can only suggest that you buy a little more than you think you'll need. At worst, you won't use all its options. At best, those options will prove to be fun and interesting and will encourage you to expand your program and reach higher.

Searching for Value

Unless your budget is already stretched to its limit, don't let price be the deciding factor in the purchase of equipment. Concentrate, instead, on getting what you pay for—value. As a doctor, I understand the problem of what I just told you to do; I'm trained in medicine, not mechanics or engineering. How would I, or anybody else not so mechanically inclined, be able to judge a complex piece of equipment? Start with the warranty. The warranty offered by a company says a lot about the value that company places on its equipment. Use this as a screening tool: compare the warranties on different makes of equipment you are considering. This includes making sure the warranty can be fulfilled. A warranty's promises are worthless if there is no one to service your product.

Such was the case with a treadmill belonging to a friend of mine. When it stopped working for no apparent reason, Eric found out that a repairman would charge $35 an hour, including traveling time, to fix it. The closest repairman was over 100 miles away. He decided to load it into his Jeep and take it there himself. "The thing had to weigh close to 400 pounds," he said (295 pounds according to its manual), and it took three people plus a lot of ingenuity just to get it into that Jeep. But the real insult came when he got it to the repair shop. They unloaded it, carried it inside, plugged it in, and turned it on. It started right away. The repairman checked the machine carefully, but it was clear that he didn't think a thing was wrong with it, and as he turned up the speed, Eric heard him mumble, "This is a nice machine."

Of course there was something wrong with the machine, but it was with the control panel rather than the motor. That diagnosis was made a week later during a telephone conversation with one of the company's troubleshooters, after the machine stopped working again. One of the beauties of home equipment is that it won't get abused by hoards of other people; it should last for years with only minor service requirements. Still, a malfunction could happen, as it did with Eric's treadmill. If a company doesn't offer service in your area, check out its troubleshooting program. A good troubleshooter is a first-rate alternative to a 200-mile drive.

Closely related to service is assembly. Assembly may be a small inconvenience when you're putting together a simple exercycle or weight bench, but with some equipment, like a multistation weight machine, it could threaten the patience of even the most mechanically inclined person. Before you buy any machine, find out what options it has for assembly. Some manufacturers include in the purchase a charge for sending someone to your home to install their equipment, and a similar service may be available from dealers who sell many brands of equipment for home use. But it may not be a bargain. Custom assembly could increase the purchase price as much as 40 percent. Consider this when you judge the value of equipment.

So much of the concept of value is decided by your attitude. Don't mislabel exercise as recreation. Recreation is a leisure activity pursued at your discretion. Exercise is *not* a discretionary activity; it is a necessary part of your life, and any equipment for it is an investment in your health and well-being. This means not that you should spend great sums of money, but that you should settle for nothing less than what you want, even with limited funds.

Checking Specific Features

There are three kinds of features: mechanics, safety, and comfort. Mechanics relates to how the machine works. Does it have a motor, and if so, what kind? Does it run rough or smooth, noisy or quiet? Safety relates to such items as handrails, pedals, foot rests, and stability. Can the machine tip over easily? Can you stop it quickly or get off safely in an emergency? The last feature is comfort. If all machines were built for the human body, comfort would be a given, and there would be no reason to mention it. But they are not—though I have no idea what body they are designed for. Before you buy any machine, try it out or at least ask someone who has, how it feels. Does it have leg room, a comfortable seat, plenty of footspace? Many machines don't. (See Figure 8.1 for a review of the factors to consider in evaluating exercise equipment.)

Figure 8.1   *EVALUATING EXERCISE EQUIPMENT*

Purpose   Is the equipment for your primary exercise or cross-training? Will you use it frequently or rarely? Buy what you *WANT*, not what you think you should.

Value   Compare warranties as an indication of a machine's reliability. Investigate the complexity of assembly; can you do it or is it worth paying someone else to put it together?

Features   Mechanics - Does it run rough or smooth? Is it noisy or quiet? Are controls and adjustments convenient?

Safety   - Is it stable or will it easily tip over? Are handrails, pedals, footrests well designed? Can you stop safely in an emergency?

Comfort   - How does it feel? Is the seat comfortable? Is there ample leg room? Does it "fit" you?

EXERCYCLE. Probably the most popular piece of equipment is the exercycle. Almost everyone is familiar with cycling, and most exercycles are quite affordable, require little floor space, and provide a completely non-impact aerobic workout. For years all exercycles were of the upright variety—the bike you rode as a child mounted on an immovable stand. Recently, however, we have seen the entry of another kind of exercycle into the market. Called a recumbent bike, it has a bigger "footprint" than the upright models, taking up more space in your home as well as in your budget. Recumbent bikes are always more expensive. Both upright and recumbent models can be manual or motorized and computerized. Some upright models have a dual action feature that allows you to pump on the handle bars while you pump on the pedals. Pumping with all limbs, you'll certainly condition your upper and lower body, but you won't be able to read, a favorite EXTRAcising activity of mine.

- *Mechanics.* Look for a bike with a smooth, quiet ride. The seat should easily adjust to multiple height settings and it should tilt backward or forward for rider comfort. When seated on the bike, you should be able to easily reach the resistance controls, with the speedometer and odometer always within clear view. In a dual-action exercycle, make sure you have the option of *not* using the handle action. There will be days when you just want to peddle.

- *Safety.* The bike should feel tight, sturdy, and stable—it should be very difficult to tip over. It should also be built for your body, particularly the length of your legs. Riding a bike that has a seat-to-peddle distance that is too long or too short for your legs stresses your knees. If the seat can't be adjusted to the right height or it can't be adjusted without a wrench—a major inconvenience when more than one person will be riding it—consider it unsafe.

- *Comfort.* When you sit on an upright model your weight is completely supported by your buttocks, so look for a comfortable seat with plenty of width and cushioning. Recumbent models are, in general, more comfortable. They distribute your weight over your back and buttocks, a valuable feature if you have lower back problems, or just don't like the upright's sitting position. On any bike, the peddles should have foot straps or toe clips. Into these your feet should slide easily, and they should be able to pull up and push down effectively during an entire revolution.

CROSS-COUNTRY SKI SIMULATOR. This is one of my favorite pieces of equipment. Great for beginners and veterans alike, a cross-country ski machine offers a wide range of exercise intensities and gives you the option of exercising your lower body only, or both your upper and lower body at the same time.

- *Mechanics.* The ski mechanism should be smooth and quiet, but not silent (that's expecting too much) and all actions independent. When you cross-country ski on snow, each foot can move independently. Therefore, a good cross-country ski simulator does not tie the motion of one foot sliding forward to the other foot sliding backward. Both skis should be able to slide simultaneously in the same direction. In the sport of cross-country skiing there is a technique called skating, pushing off on one foot, while sliding the other forward—without using the poles. Can the machine simulate this? It can if its poling device is not, in anyway, connected with the skis. This is an important option. It gives you the freedom to work your lower body only. Other options such as an attached pulse monitor or an apparatus that allows you to elevate the front end of the machine for skiing uphill are handy, but not worth much extra cost. You can always elevate the machine with a block of wood and, as for the pulse monitor, it's more useful if it's not attached. What you must have is an easy-to-read distance gauge and speedometer and an easy-to-adjust resistance control.

- *Safety.* Cross-country ski machines are typically light, so inspect it for stability. Even during a rigorous workout it should sit solidly on the floor without any rocking.

- *Comfort.* Not only are people different heights, they have different builds. A hip rest should accommodate this by adjusting vertically and pivoting. During long workouts you'll appreciate one that's well cushioned, yet firm.

STAIRCLIMBER. Stairclimbers build. They build your cardiovascular system, they build your quadriceps, they build your calves, they build just about every muscle below your waist. And all this building is impact free. By removing the noxious downstairs portion of stairclimbing—those who climb up don't have to come down—stairclimbers provide a vigorous, but safe workout. They also take up little space. But stairclimbers aren't cheap. A good one costs more than an exercycle or cross-country ski machine.

- *Mechanics.* During any kind of aerobic exercise you never want to continuously rely on one leg more than the other. Therefore, insist on a stairclimber with an independent step mechanism—one foot doesn't have to go up while the other goes down—and a smooth motion; both features make it harder for you to favor one side. Also insist on a stairclimber that allows you to change speed and resistance while you're exercising. Some models force you to get off to make these adjustments, which can spoil your workout. Another workout spoiler is a monitor that is inconvenient to read—you can't get a reading of speed or the number of flights without pushing enough buttons to reach the moon.

- *Safety.* By definition, stair climbing requires you to leave floor level, and stairclimbers must be built for this. One of the features you generally pay more for is the weight necessary to make a stairclimber stable. Don't skimp on stability. A rickety machine can tip over, putting you physically at risk. But even a machine that sits solidly on the floor can be unsafe. A safe stairclimber must also have well-placed handrails to hold onto for balance when necessary and large pedals that remain parallel to the floor no matter where you place your foot.

- *Comfort.* Pedal size and placement will influence your comfort the most. Because your balance is constantly shifting as you climb stairs, wide pedals a comfortable distance apart are needed to give you freedom to move normally. But large pedals do more than help you keep your balance. They allow for many different foot placements—for example, the toes over the front edge or the heels over the back edge or both squarely on the pedal—which make it possible to work different lower leg muscles.

ROWER. In the late 1980s, sales of rowing machines surged, but for the last several years their tide has receded. The likely reason is that other kinds of exercise equipment flooded the market, taking away some of their sales. Yet rowing was and still is a good exercise. Shopping for a rowing machine, you will find two versions: those with hydraulic resistance and those with flywheel resistance.

- *Mechanics.* Flywheel rowers are more realistic in their movement, but they are more costly in terms of the space they require and the prices they demand. Realistic movement or not, both kinds of rowers will give you a good workout if they run smoothly. The curse of any exercise equipment is that it doesn't, and a chattering, vibrating 20- or 30-minute row will exercise your patience. So will noise. With their loud history, the flywheel models are more suspect of this flaw than their hydraulic competitors. But today all good quality machines should run reasonably quiet.

- *Safety.* The major safety issue with rowing is the exercise itself. A rowing mechanism with inconsistent resistance—it becomes easier or harder somewhere in the rowing motion—is a recipe for an injury. To avoid injury, you *must* have a smooth, consistent tension throughout. Leg room is another safety issue. If the seat doesn't slide far enough, your legs won't be able to fully extend, forcing you to stay in an unnatural cramped position throughout the rowing motion, another recipe that cooks up an injury. A third caution is to avoid machines that don't have adjustable foot rests with straps to hold your feet in place. Besides enabling your legs to work in both directions, the straps stabilize your body during the exercise. They hold you in the motion, which is where you want to be. But the back injuries that rowing machines are renowned for causing can happen even with the best-designed equipment. Here the villain is posture; look for a rowing machine with a seat that has lower back support.

- *Comfort.* While rowing, your weight is concentrated on your buttocks and lower back. Add the pushing force of your legs and you put even more weight on those areas. Hence a well-designed seat with ample padding is a must. A footrest that pivots as you move through the stroke also adds to your comfort; it gives the exercise a more natural feel and during a workout of many strokes this makes a big difference. Always check for this feature, as many models don't have it.

TREADMILL. Once sold only to commercial gyms, treadmills for home use are now made by many companies. That these home models are not built for heavy and sometimes abusive use the professional ones must bear is not a sign of poor quality; in their capacity, they are just as dependable. Home treadmills can be motorized or manual. The manual models are adequate for walking but not for running. Having to push the belt with that much force, you stress your lower body, especially your joints. This is a serious limitation. The motorized treadmills are good for both walking and running, which is why I recommend them.

- *Mechanics.* The motor of any treadmill should not be less than 1.5 horsepower (on a continuous duty rating); smaller than that and it won't generate enough speed for running. But you don't need too much speed either. A motor that generates over 10 miles per hour is overkill and probably overpriced too. Aside from horsepower, motors also vary in the kind of current they use. Alternating current (AC) motors run at a constant speed. For you to walk or run at variable speeds the belt speed must be controlled by some sort of mechanical means, which can be troublesome. Choose, instead, a treadmill with a direct current (DC) motor, which runs at variable speeds allowing the belt speed to be controlled directly by the motor. DC-powered treadmills run smoother, and when turned on they will restart at the minimum speed, not at whatever speed the machine was last on, as with AC models. Some treadmills have an incline feature to mimic hills. For runners this is a leg sparing feature; it gives you the intensity of uphill running but none of the pounding of downhill running. Just make sure it's easy to make this adjustment on the machine.

- *Safety.* Any motorized treadmill needs adequate space behind it in case you slip and fall. The length of its belt should depend on what you use the machine for: the faster you run, the longer the belt you need. As for its width, nobody runs in a perfectly straight line. A belt has to be wide enough to accommodate some weaving. The next two features—sturdy handrails and easy-to-reach on-off controls—saved my friend Eric from injury. Eric ran indoors and outdoors. When running outdoors, he always took Eddie, his German Shepherd, along. One day Eddie decided he wanted to run with him indoors too, and he suddenly jumped on the treadmill while Eric was logging in a 4-mile run. In the seconds that followed, confusion reigned: a man and a dog struggled to regain their balance. Fortunately, Eric was able to grab onto a handrail with one hand and shut the machine off with a swing of the other. Neither man nor dog were hurt. But Eddie never went near the running machine again.

- *Comfort.* Treadmills are much kinder to your joints than pavement, and the newer models have even more cushioning. This is an important option because it lessens the harsh impact of running. Don't pass up this joint insurance.

MULTISTATION WEIGHT MACHINE. A multistation weight machine is a single machine with several stations at which you can do a number of weight-lifting exercises. There are many such machines on the market. Some are useless. But don't rely on price to tell you which ones; there are some very expensive and useless machines out there. And don't go by what's being used at commercial gyms either. Nowadays these gyms are switching to circuits of single machines that each work a specific muscle group. For a gym it's a good investment. For a homeowner, however, it's not practical. Excellent as these machines are for building strength and endurance, they take up a lot of space and are very expensive, so consider only a multistation model. Inexpensive machines have significant limitations, while expensive ones can be loaded with unnecessary options and require too much floor space: add to the size of the machine itself the space needed for access to all weight-lifting stations around its perimeter. Even if price and space aren't factors in your purchase decision, one question should always stand out in your mind: can I conveniently do a *total body* workout on this machine? If the answer is no, don't buy it.

- *Mechanics.* Inexpensive machines use hydraulic pistons, flexible rods, rubber bands, and other odd ways of generating resistance, and they are often hard to adjust and impossible to measure. Never are these bargain machines a bargain. Shop, instead, for the classic system of stacked weights with cables and pulleys; it will give you a smoother, more uniform action. Always note the least amount of weight you can add. If it's 10 pounds, it's too much; a woman should never increase weight by that amount, and depending on the exercise and strength involved, many men shouldn't either.

- *Safety.* Another warning about the cheaper machines: many don't supply resistance in both directions. Instead, the resistance is only in lifting; lowering is a freefall adventure. Nothing could be more dangerous. That is nothing but an unstable machine. Again we're visiting bargain-town, where the machines tend to be unstable and must therefore be assembled against a wall or another piece of equipment. Would you want to "lift weights" on this? Invest in a more expensive free-standing machine.

- *Comfort.* Not all machines, including some of the more expensive ones, are built for a smaller body frame. Make sure your body fits the machine for all the exercises you want to do. No one wants to contort himself or spend precious minutes making changes and adjustments to the equipment just to do a particular exercise. (See Figure 8.2 for a summary of equipment features to look for.)

FREE WEIGHTS AND OTHER EQUIPMENT. Like a well-designed multistation machine, free weights can give you an excellent total body workout. Figure 8.3 compares a multistation workout with a free-weight workout. For a free-weight workout that is almost as convenient as a multistation one, all you need is a sturdy weight lifting bench and two sets of iron weights. I suggest two sets of weights because it saves you time in assembling barbells and dumbbells for different exercises and still costs nothing compared to a quality machine. Free weights also save space. Unlike a machine, they can be stored economically. I know someone who stored them under her bed and just rolled them out to exercise. She also "stored" her weight bench. When it was time to exercise, out from a dark corner of her bedroom it came; it was that light and easy to move. From this story you know that some benches are very simple. Some, however, are so complicated they resemble lower-priced weight machines without the weights. What kind do you need for a total body workout? Only a simple one with a knee extension attachment. But check it for stability. I once tipped a bench over when I sat on the wrong side with heavy dumbbells in my hand. It was a surprise I didn't need.

Off the beaten jogging path that leads to the more popular exercise machines are other worthwhile machines you might consider including in your home gym. One of these is a ladderclimber. Similar to a stairclimber, ladderclimbers also have an attachment that works the upper body. It's a machine that will give you a total body

Figure 8.2 EQUIPMENT FEATURES TO LOOK FOR

	Mechanics	Safety	Comfort
Exercycle	Smooth, quiet ride. Option of not using handlebar action (if any) and peddling at the same time.	Tight, sturdy, and stable. Difficult to tip over. Seat-to-peddle distance easy to adjust.	Comfortable wide, cushioned seat. Consider recumbent model. Foot straps or toe clips.
CC Skier	Independent ski action. Smooth and relatively quiet. Option of not using poling device.	Stability from tipping over or rocking. Adjustable incline without significant loss of stability.	Well-cushioned hip rest with vertical and pivoting adjustability. Well-fitting "binding" for comfortable shoe.
Stairclimber	Independent step mechanism. Smooth motion. Convenient to change speed and resistance.	Stability of utmost importance since you must leave the floor level. Well-placed handrails.	Comfortable pedal size and placement to feel balanced as you constantly shift your weight.
Rower	Flywheel type is more realistic but costlier than hydraulic. Either should be quiet and free from vibration.	Consistent tension and resistance throughout complete rowing motion. Adequate leg room on full extension.	Padded seat with lower back support. Pivoting foot rest as you move through the stroke provides natural motion.
Treadmill	Direct current (DC) motor optimal. Ten mph maximum speed needed. Easy to adjust elevation feature, if any.	Belt length and width must accommodate your running style. Well-placed handrails and easy-to-reach off switch.	Cushioning technology incorporated into running surface to lessen impact. Easy-to-reach controls.
Multistation Weight Machine	Avoid hydraulic pistons, flexible rods and rubber bands. Choose smooth acting stacked weights with cables and pulleys.	Must supply resistance in both directions. Free-standing unit preferable but must have excellent stability.	Machine built to fit your body frame without requiring tedious adjustments. Must have ample space to use stations properly.

Figure 8.3   **EQUIVALENT WEIGHT LIFTING EXERCISES**

	Free Weights	**Machines**
Back	Reverse flies One-arm rowing	Seated rowing Lat pulldown
Chest	Supine flies Bench press Front lifts	Seated or vertical butterfly Chest press Upright rowing
Shoulders	Front lifts Side lifts (lateral arm raises)	Upright rowing Upright rowing
Legs	Reverse leg lifts Weighted leg extensions Heel raises	Knee or leg curl Leg extensions Seated or standing calf raises
Arms	Dumbbell curls Triceps barbell curls Kickbacks	Biceps curls Pulley push downs Triceps press downs, triceps extensions

Note: Although all exercises are not identical, they will work the same muscle groups.

---

workout. Far less expensive, but much more portable is the slide-board. This innovative, but simple apparatus gives you a vigorous, low-impact workout at home and on the road. My final recommendation goes to a chinning bar. No piece of equipment is as simple and yet so useful. Depending on the position of your head and hands, you can use it to build strength in your shoulders, arms, chest, and back. Just anchor it securely enough to support your weight.

SMART SHOPPING TIPS

Now that you know what to look for in exercise equipment, your next problem is to decide who to buy from. Should you buy from a department store or a general sporting goods store, a mail order catalog or an exercise equipment store? Or perhaps it would be better to buy from the manufacturer.

Department Stores

One problem with department stores and general sporting goods stores is that they are in the business of selling a wide range of products, and they can't afford to educate their salespeople about complex equipment like exercise machines. Even knowing exactly what questions to ask is not good enough. You had better know all the answers too because the salespeople won't. Not that ignorance will stop some of them from talking. From the stories I've heard, it's obvious that some people live by the motto, "If it sounds good, it's okay to say." Well it doesn't always sound good, and it's not okay to say. But I have more experience than most shoppers do at recognizing that.

Another problem is that these stores usually carry a limited number of models, some of them outdated. Why choose from a small sample when you can compare a wide variety? What's more, these stores rarely offer assembly and do not assist with service other than to refer you to the manufacturer.

Mail Order

Mail order catalogs generally have a wider selection than department stores, but they also have the same problem with inexperienced salespeople and no assembly or service. If you buy from a catalog company that sells fitness equipment—not a shoe catalog that offers just a few such items—your chances of getting what you want are better. Of course you'll still have to deal with the problem of assembly. But don't assume that you *must* assemble it yourself. Depending on the item, some companies will assemble it—for a charge. There is no such thing as free assembly.

Manufacturers

Some equipment you can buy directly from the manufacturer. Here the knowledge problem is just the opposite of the department store's or mail order's. Often the manufacturer's salespeople know so much that they lose you as they ramble on, raising their machine to the lofty heights of exercise elites while simultaneously slam dunking every other model on the market. Be prepared to separate the hype from the fact. That includes the videos many manufacturers will offer to send you. One video I watched made the exercise machine seem like God's answer to fitness, designed to easily fold up and be stored in a closet. As it turned out, the primary exercise you got from the machine was trying to fold it up and carry it to a closet—which I couldn't do. Yet the woman in the video could. In fact she effortlessly picked it up and carried it under one arm into the closet. Who was that woman? And what closet is that empty?

Reputable firms have truly knowledgeable people who can help you with the specifications you need. They can also guide you in making repairs by troubleshooting over the phone, and if that doesn't work, they'll have you send the malfunctioning part to them for repair. This may not be the most convenient service system, but it does work. If you suspect the reliability of a particular model—perhaps your research uncovered a potential problem—or you live in the "country" where service is not readily available, upgrade to a higher-quality model. What you're paying for is extra reliability and it's worth it.

Specialty Stores

A specialty store that sells exercise equipment only is the most convenient outlet to buy from. But before you visit one, call and ask them to send you reading material on the equipment you're considering. Then visit the showroom. There you can usually try out different models, comparing one manufacturer's to another's while a knowledgeable salesperson stands by for questions. No other vendor can offer this. Nor can other vendors usually offer home delivery with assembly and a service department for maintenance and repairs. Many specialty stores do—though it's always a good idea to make sure these services are available. Still, the extra service and convenience aren't free. You must decide whether they're worth the higher price. (See Figure 8.4 to review your shopping alternatives.)

FINDING A HOME FOR YOUR NEW GYM

My first home gym was in the basement. It had a NordicTrack® cross-country ski machine, a Tunturi® exercycle, a weight bench, and a mixed array of old weights handed down to me from my brother. Next to the NordicTrack® were homemade wooden shelves

Figure 8.4	**TO BUY OR NOT TO BUY?**	
	Yes	**No**
Department Store	... if you know exactly what you want, it's reliable, and you're willing to assemble it.	... if you need guidance from a salesperson, specifications, and options.
Mail Order	... if you know enough about the product and are satisfied with the selection, reliability, and price.	... if your only source of information is the picture and write-up in the catalog or if assembly is complex.
Manufacturer	... if you don't need to compare with other makes, are certain of its reliability or you have no other source.	... if you don't want to assemble it or suspect repair service may be inconvenient.
Specialty Store	... if you need experience to evaluate your needs, explain equipment's use, customize it, or assemble it.	... if you don't perceive sufficient value for the higher price you'll likely be charged.

that held a lamp, a tape player, and some reading material. On the floor was a large fan to cool me as I skied and cycled. It was exercise heaven: private, functional, and just a flight of stairs away. What used to be a dark, dusty, dungeon of a room, used mainly to store Christmas decorations, old books, and dishes, was now the most important place in the house. The basement was the most convenient room to put equipment; it had extra space, electrical outlets, and heat, and by using it, I didn't have to give up other valuable space, like my study or the guest bedroom so well used during holidays.

At the other extreme is adding another room on your house. A good blueprint should include lighting, cooling, ventilation, noise control, and electrical outlets—plus extra structural support and ceiling height. My first pieces of equipment didn't require electricity, but the light, the fan, and the tape player did. One person I know planned to use his attic, only to find out that he needed to have the attic floor reinforced because it had been built to function only as a ceiling. For a more open, airy feel, plan plenty of windows and add mirrors. Mirrors will not only give the illusion of more space, they will make it possible to check your form as you lift weights.

Your gym could be quite simple, consisting of a small weight bench, some free weights, and an exercycle, but no two pieces of equipment have to be in the same room. What constitutes a home gym is exercise equipment kept anywhere in your home. If a space problem makes it impossible to keep all your equipment in one room, spread it around. A weight bench can be tucked away in almost any room. But beware of fold-away equipment. The exercise industry, aware that most people have a space problem, has invented some ingenious folding machines—that is, they're ingenious sounding in the sales brochure. At home they are inconvenient, if not impossible, to use. Even if the equipment does fold and store as claimed, how much time and effort does the folding and storing take? Too much. Usually this "effort and folding" option demands much strength and persistence, and the folded equipment more room than any nook or cranny has to fit it. Don't be fooled by this miracle option. Matter does not fold away or disappear. Always place your equipment where you have instant access to it.

Next, consider who will be using the gym. Will your spouse or friends join you in a vigorous workout? A gym that can accommodate several exercisers at once is an advantage; it promotes group exercise, which many people consider more fun than exercising alone because it transplants the social aspect of fitness clubs right into your home. So invite your friends and thank them for their good company by giving them the opportunity to work out on quality equipment. Make your gym the showcase of your house. Good exercise equipment may not look like works of art, but it does look expensive and well made and will inform anyone with decent vision that you mean business. If people tend to gravitate to the same piece of equipment, add a second one to your gym. Duplicates of equipment save time and add to the party atmosphere. When two people exercise together on two exercycles, or two slideboards, or two cross-country ski machines, or two rowing machines, it heightens the spirit of friendship. They're both literally in the same boat.

Whichever style of home gym you decide on—large or small, elaborate or simple—make it as warm and inviting as possible, even when you are not exercising. Add comfortable furniture and attractive accessories; in short add your personal signature. Making your fitness room home makes take-home fitness fun.

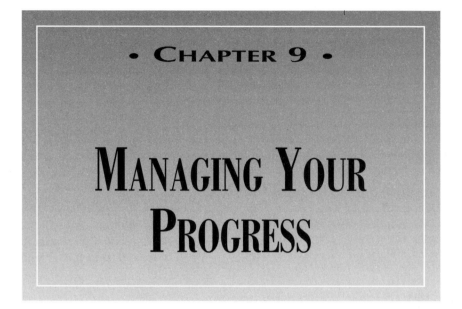

CHAPTER 9

MANAGING YOUR PROGRESS

All this talk about designing a fitness program brings us to the important, but often overlooked, area of managing your progress. How are you going to keep score? And why should you bother to?

Imagine you are on a firing range, shooting at a target that happens to be your ultimate fitness goal. If you hit a bull's-eye, you are instantly transformed into the fitness idol of your dreams—the Jean-Claude Van Damme of your company, the Jackie Joyner-Kersee of your division. You know how to shoot; the previous chapters have taught you that. But now on the firing range you're not sure how you did—you can't see if you hit the bull's-eye and you'll change into your fitness idol only if you *know* that you did. Are you going to sit there and wonder about it? Or are you going to run up to that target to see if there's a bullet hole that will make you Jean-Claude or Jackie?

RECOGNIZING PROGRESS CANNOT BE TAKEN FOR GRANTED

Recall the three principles of the goal-reward circle in Chapter 2: set a goal, accomplish it, reward yourself. The goal in that circle must be specific and challenging, yet reachable within a reasonable time;

in short, realistic and valuable. By achieving the goal, you stimulate your reward pathway, which responds by giving you a pleasant feeling of satisfaction. This pleasant feeling is an intrinsic reward. To it add an extrinsic reward—something of value that you give yourself—inciting your reward pathway to emit another pleasant feeling. Not once, but twice, you are rewarded for reaching a goal. This double-pronged positive feedback system is why goals are so vital to success.

That your reward pathway responds so well to goal accomplishment does not mean that it's in charge of everything. If you form a goal, your reward pathway won't remember it. Nor will it keep track of your progress toward that goal. Consider your goal a destination. It's your job to think about it, to visualize what it will look like, to watch for guideposts on the way, and to recognize it when you get there.

Many people get lost on the way. They start out in the right direction with an excellent goal. Then time passes, and they not only forget what their goal was, they forget where they started, washing out all evidence of progress and shattering their goal-reward circle. Some of these people almost reach their goals. Some actually do reach them. But none feel the triumph and excitement—it all happened too gradually. As a psychiatrist, one of the most astonishing things I learned about human nature is how seldom people give themselves credit for their accomplishments.

The example of target practice makes this point clearly. You can have the finest target, clearly drawn and easy to see from a distance. You can have the most accurate firearm and the best shooting technique. But you won't have the satisfaction of knowing how well you shot, unless you see the bullet holes, proof that you hit the target. I chose target practice as an example because I learned an explicit lesson about feedback on the target range. One day several years ago, I was at an Army target range, trying to qualify as a Marksman. I had been practicing and gaining accuracy for a week. But on that day I couldn't seem to knock the target over even once, and with each shot I became more frustrated and negative. "Why did I even care about qualifying as a Marksman?" I asked myself. Finally, in total disgust, I walked over to the target and found that it was so full of bullet holes it no longer had enough substance to be knocked over by the momentum of the bullets hitting it. Of course some of my bullets had hit it, but I hadn't seen the target spring backward. It felt the same as if I had missed.

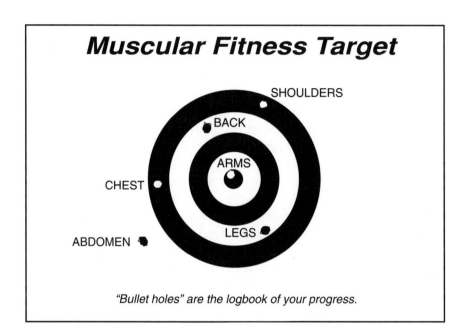

Muscular Fitness Target

"Bullet holes" are the logbook of your progress.

A LOGBOOK IS YOUR EXERCISE AUTOBIOGRAPHY

Don't let what happened to me on the target range happen to you in your fitness program. Serve notice to yourself when you accomplish something; write your exercise autobiography. Most of us have reams of experience at this. How many annual reports, or analyses of business trends, or budgets or sales projections have you prepared? And you keep records at home too. Would you write a check without noting it in your checkbook or throw away your bank statements? No—you want proof of how you are spending your money.

Still, you've probably never created a record as personal as an exercise autobiography. So start slowly by setting up a simple logbook that tracks one kind of exercise, probably your whole program at first. As your program evolves, your exercise logbook should evolve to reflect it. What used to be enough detail—say, a notation that you jogged 15 minutes on a particular date—will no longer suffice: you've added speedwork for the racing season, cycling for cross-training, weight lifting for your upper body, and all the goals connected with these exercises.

Besides being a constant reminder of your goals, a logbook creates a compass that guides you in the right direction. By reminding you where you are, it keeps you moving forward. Your logbook will tell you how many kilometers you rowed yesterday. It will tell you how many sit-ups you did last Thursday. Reading this, you might get insulted. Surely you can remember how many sit-ups you did—and you probably could if your program were static: the same workout day after day. But no one's program should be static.

To say that you can remember everything about your program is to say that you can remember everything. Can you remember everything you ate yesterday, or the day before? Diet researchers have long known that food diaries prepared at the end of each day are inaccurate, a factor they must work around when compiling their data and arriving at conclusions. Not even a well-organized person can keep a totally accurate food diary.

Speaking as a well-organized person who has the added advantage of being trained to notice subtle mental and physical shifts in patients, I know I couldn't keep track of the changes in my program if I didn't write things down. I once became discouraged about my weight lifting. It seemed I wasn't making progress with my bench presses; I was doing the same repetitions with the same weight for over a month. But my logbook told me another story. It said I was pressing the same weight for only three workouts—a little over a week. It also reminded me that I had recently increased my repetitions in another exercise, barbell curls. The moral of this story: no matter how well-organized you are, you can't recognize everything that's going on in a multifaceted fitness program.

Obviously my feeling stalled at weight lifting was related to my mood at the time. A logbook, though it may contain emotional remarks, gives you the hard facts. For example, if you have an "off" workout, when you can't accomplish what you had in the past—

your time was unusually slow or your repetitions fell short—your logbook would point out that it's just a bad day and in no way indicative of your ability. Your logbook is also just as likely to capture a good day. Such days shine out of it, showing you what you're capable of, motivating you to reach for higher goals.

A logbook is a record of your fitness successes. It announces when you reach your goals, spinning you around another revolution of the goal-reward circle. All of us need this encouragement; our reward pathways thrive on it. Beyond that, there's the extrinsic reward you promised yourself when you set the goal and it makes your reward pathway even happier. As you complete several goal-reward circles, you gain momentum. Your accomplishments build your confidence. Your confidence spurs you to achieve more. It becomes a cycle. But the cycle can continue only if you feed it the progress you harvest from your exercise logbook (see Figure 9.1).

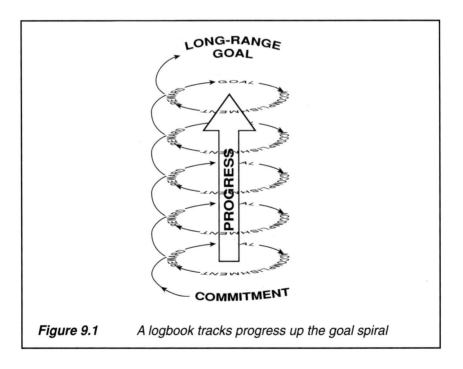

Figure 9.1   *A logbook tracks progress up the goal spiral*

A Logbook Is Also Your Coach and Doctor

Trust your logbook as you would trust your coach or doctor; it's as dependable and in some cases more knowledgeable. Your doctor can diagnose a muscle pull or stress fracture. But he or she can't tell you exactly why the injury happened. Perhaps a new pair of shoes, though theoretically correct for your feet, leaves your ankles and knees aching. In the examination room, the topic of shoes may never come up. In your logbook, a note of a shoe change—an important detail because shoes are your first line of defense against impact—will stand out for review. Your logbook can also tell you when you've exceeded the exercise guidelines of this book: you'll read that your knees always ache after you increase the tension (too much) on your exercycle or that your back hurts after you double up on a cross-country skiing workout. It even knows when your doctor is wrong. Three orthopedic surgeons told me that bike riding was excellent for my knees; it was a nonweight-bearing exercise that would build my quadriceps, the muscles most capable of stabilizing my knee caps. That made sense. What didn't make sense was the continued pain and swelling of my knees. Finally I looked at my logbook and confirmed my suspicions: cycling consistently aggravated my knees. When I discovered cross-country skiing, relegating cycling to an every-so-often cross-training exercise, my knees improved dramatically.

Listen to your body. If you have a trouble spot, perhaps fragile knees or a sensitive back, note what irritates it. Describe the workout that taxes it, recording what pushes you to the edge. Describe the workout that left you pain free and fresh. Write in your logbook a story of your limits, and then reread it so you know that there are boundaries to gently push outward, not blockades over which to vault into an injury or setback.

Sometimes exercisers do vault over their limits and injure themselves. If you do, use your logbook as a guide to recovery, especially if it's an injury you have had before. What did you do, for example, the last time your back acted up? Did you apply moist heat? Did you replace running with cycling for a while or do sit-ups? A friend traveling on business injured his back by grabbing a suitcase he thought was light but turned out to be as heavy as six bowling balls. Two years later his back suffered again when his 70-

pound Collie playfully pounced on him. But this time he had a written guide of what to do: how long to completely rest his back and what exercises to safely do while still healing. Like the doctor who had seen a thousand of these injuries before, his logbook knew exactly how to treat it.

So did mine. One morning in a fit of impatience, I decided to do my regular workout in half its normal time. The result of that blistering session was a sore left knee that took weeks to heal with my hit-and-miss therapy. Eight months later when the same knee pain came back, my logbook was ready. Reading it I not only realized the cause, I knew the stretching therapy that finally healed it. The pain that could have lasted for weeks, disappeared in days. Injuries, whether they are caused by overzealous exercise or not, can happen from time to time. Let your logbook expertly guide you away from the confusion and worry.

Expert guidance is a commodity highly valued by professional athletes; hence a good coach is worth his weight in endorsements. A good coach knows how hard to work an athlete. By watching an athlete work, a coach can suggest changes in his training routine that develops his full potential. But the line between reaching his full potential and overworking himself is a fine one. A coach must find it through careful trial and error. Your logbook can do the same job. It records your trials and errors, shows you your limits, and gives you ideas for changing your workouts.

HOW TO DESIGN A LOGBOOK

What should your logbook look like? Should each page be neatly divided into subsections or just be a blank piece of paper awaiting your spontaneous scribble? There is no pat answer. Logbooks can be as different as the individuals who create them, but mainly they will fall into two classes: free-form logbooks or programmed logbooks.

Getting Started

As the examples in Figure 9.2 show, a free-form logbook is little more than a blank page with a date. On it you note what exercises you did and anything that indicates for how long and at what inten-

---

Figure 9.2	**FREE-FORM LOGBOOK - Sample 1**

Date: Goal:

Cardio:
_____
_____
_____

Muscular:
_____
_____

Comments:
_____
_____
_____

FREE-FORM LOGBOOK - Sample 2

		Cardio			Muscular		
Date	Type	Time	Heart Rate	Type	Weight	Sets/ Reps	Flexi- bility

sity you worked—time, heart rate, reps. Usually beginners start out with a free-form logbook. You are busy shaping your program, experimenting with different exercises, juggling schedules to add workouts, and looking into fitness centers and home equipment.

Then as your program evolves, your logbook evolves. When you arrive at a stable exercise routine, a programmed logbook similar to that in Figure 9.3 will probably be more convenient. This is

---

Figure 9.3   ***PROGRAMMED LOGBOOK SAMPLE***

Date:

CARDIO   Target Heart Rate:

☐ 2-Mile Run   Weather
   Time: Temperature:
   Heart Rate: Other:
   Observations & Feelings:

MUSCULAR   Goal:

☐ Supine flies   ☐ Side lifts
   Set 1 reps   Set 1 reps
   Set 2 reps   Set 2 reps

☐ Barbell bench press   ☐ Reverse flies
   Set 1 reps   Set 1 reps
   Set 2 reps   Set 2 reps

☐ Front lifts   ☐ One-arm rowing
   Set 1 reps   Set 1 reps
   Set 2 reps   Set 2 reps

Note: Allow 30 seconds between sets.

STRETCHING   Hold for 30 seconds

☐ Hamstrings   ☐ Upper back   ☐ Neck   ☐ Quadriceps

☐ Lower back   ☐ Chest   ☐ Hips

---

especially true of exercise programs that include weight lifting, with its multitude of exercises, which are further complicated by changing poundage and the number of repetitions and sets you do for each. For most weight lifters it is more convenient to list exercises in advance, filling in the pounds, reps, and sets as they go along. On Mondays and Wednesdays, for example, you could list the exercises for the arms, back, and chest. On Tuesdays and Thursdays, list the ones that concentrate on the abdomen and lower body. The advantage here is that your logbook reminds you of what you planned to do, literally pulling you toward your goals. The drawback is that it's somewhat inflexible. It takes time for you to arrive at a stable routine, and even then you will change it to challenge boredom, to accommodate special circumstances such as busy times at work and to steer you toward new goals.

Make It Easy to Read

Eventually you may come full circle and again use a free-form logbook. But by this time it's more convenient because you are much more experienced and have probably developed a personal shorthand for describing what you do.

Convenience, then, is a factor you must consider when designing your logbook. Don't have one section in your logbook for cardio fitness, another for strength and still another for stretching. You'll be forever flipping through pages to get to this section, making a daily entry in one while forgetting to make it in another—driving yourself crazy. Keep everything you do on one day on the same page.

That brings us to the page size. If your entire workout has to fit on one page, a 2 $1/2''$ by 5'' pad won't do. Remember, the purpose of a logbook is to give you feedback. It can do that only if you record the information in it first. A small logbook with tiny writing and no detail feeds little back to you—it doesn't have the data necessary to answer questions and is impossible to read at a glance. Start with an 8 $1/2''$ by 11'' page. With enough experience, you may design a system that allows you to use a smaller page but don't shrink it too much.

Some suggested details to put on each page include the following:

- Date and time of day
- Kind of exercise
- Duration (time and/or distance)
- Intensity
    Poundage, reps, sets (weight lifting)
    Heart rate (cardio)

• Feelings and specific observations

Date and Time of Day

Listed first is the date and time of day. Don't assume that you'll remember the dates you exercised—weeks, months, or even years from now what could have been a very revealing statistic will be gone forever.

Another revealing statistic is the time of day. What time you exercise, often affects your reaction to it. You might notice that a morning workout starts your day better, or that a brisk midday walk or jog suits your schedule and disposition best, or that an evening workout helps you unwind after a hectic day at work. Pay attention to these preferences. They are governed by the body's circadian rhythms—physiological fluxes related to the 24-hour cycles of the Earth's rotation.

Kind of Exercise

Next, what kind of exercise did you do? Granted, that's easy enough to remember if you do only one kind of exercise, but will it be easy to remember a year or two from now after you've expanded your program with cross-training exercises or even switched to another main exercise? And if you expand your program to include a muscular fitness goal, you'll not only list each exercise along with its poundage, repetitions, and sets, you'll list them in the order in which you did them. The order can explain your progress in each. During the later exercises, your muscles will be more fatigued, decreasing the number of repetitions you are able to do.

Most exercisers won't even mention stretching in their logbooks. To them stretching amounts to a hasty afterthought and is seldom done with any consistency. Yet flexibility addresses all parts of the body. It burns calories, tones muscles, relieves stress, as well as many minor ailments like neck pain, lower back pain, arthritic pain, and general stiffness. List the stretches you do and the number of seconds you hold each of them. Flexibility can help you reach any fitness goal, but you'll never make that connection if you don't include it in your logbook. A multifaceted fitness program that includes cardio, muscular, and flexibility exercises is something to be proud of. A logbook that records those exercises keeps that pride fresh.

Duration

Another detail worth noting is the time you spent exercising. Cardio exercisers would aim for a minimum of 20 minutes a workout—because that's how long it takes for the heart to benefit—and they would also note the distance they traveled in that time. Distance adds depth to your information. Together with the time, it gives you a good idea of your exercise intensity.

Intensity

For weight lifters, record the weight you lift, the repetitions, the sets, and the time interval between sets. Of the weight lifters I know, most keep track of the pounds they're lifting—few ever bother to note the time intervals between sets. They see no reason to because they consistently use 30- or 60-second intervals and have no trouble remembering it. But a time interval shortened is an exercise intensified—without going through the trouble of loading more weight onto the bar. One small notation can accrue a big convenience.

For cardio exercise the most accurate marker of exercise intensity is heart rate. It's the gauge that tells you if you're strengthening your cardiovascular system. Some exercisers come to recognize what intensity they're working at without checking their heart rates. If you're a beginner, however, you should track your heart rate diligently. But even when you become more experienced and push your heart rate higher for greater cardio fitness, keep recording it. Noting your heart rate, you prove to yourself that you're moving closer to your goal of cardio fitness. Don't rob yourself of that proof.

But heart rate is more than just a cardio fitness gauge; it's also your comfort gauge. Compare your heart rate with your feelings and observations. An unpleasant workout could indicate that your heart rate was too high; you exceeded the limits of your conditioning and should ease up so you can enjoy your workouts again. An unusually easy workout might mean just the opposite: your heart rate was too low to move you closer to your cardio fitness goal. Tracking your heart rate isn't the easiest thing to do, yet it's well worth the trouble. From it you get an exercise barometer that's hard to beat.

Feelings and Specific Observations

The exercise barometer wouldn't, however, be quite as useful without feelings and specific observations. Too high a heart rate might not be noticed without the comment "lousy workout." A string of workouts too intense might end in injury without the warning that you feel "washed out" after them. How did you feel during your workout and what did you think of it afterward? These are the comments that coach and doctor you—that guide you away from injury and toward your goal.

Here I'm not suggesting you write a short story about every workout. Any comment summarizing your experience will do: "legs tired today," "started tired, finished strong," "felt optimistic and energetic." Some exercisers will write more, their style being naturally wordy. Others will have more to write when the workout warrants special description or explanation. But you don't need an unusual workout as a reason to write more. Adding a little "color" to your comments never hurts. The weather, your allergies, your day at work, what you ate before and after the workout—these are all the details that can lead to a self-revelation.

One such revelation happened to Karen, a lawyer and runner who, like myself, always seemed to be cold. If you asked her about winter, she would portray herself as a victim, her hands and feet constantly tortured by the cold. But when it came to running, Karen would be out there in any weather, including minus 4 degrees Fahrenheit, with a wind-chill factor of minus 42. Hearing about that frigid feat, I asked her how her hands (and feet) survived. She honestly didn't know—until she checked her logbook. It told her that running in the cold didn't bother her, that her hands and feet didn't even get cold. "And all this time I assumed it was killing me," she said. Now Karen would much rather run in the cold than the heat. There's no way to escape an "outdoor sauna."

Knowing how to exercise comfortably in cold weather depends much on what you wear. Don't guess what will be comfortable. Know exactly how many layers you'll need because your logbook includes weather conditions and the outfits that match them.

Jumping to another season, summer, we have the opposite conditions of hot, muggy, "outdoor sauna" weather. Although prop-

er dress also affects your workout—bare skin absorbs more heat—
the crucial factor is how much you drink. All the weight you lose
during exercise is water you sweat and breathe out. If you fail to
replace it by drinking before, during, and immediately after a workout, you become dehydrated, leaving yourself tired and more vulnerable to illness. Keep your logbook informed. Write down what
you weigh before and after a hot workout. The difference is the
weight of the fluids you must replace.

By jotting down your feelings you create a trail. When did you
stop enjoying your workouts? What were you doing when you felt
so strong and enthusiastic? Often the mystery is solved by your comments.

This is a chapter of suggestions, not rules. A logbook is a personal account of your experiences, and it should be designed to
include anything you want, anywhere you want it. But if there is
one rule I want to leave with you, it's this: whenever you're not sure
whether to include something in your logbook, go ahead and write
it down. Sometimes the oddest bits of information make the biggest
difference.

SEE THE BIG PICTURE

A logbook gives you more than specific feedback; it also gives you
a bigger picture by highlighting your gradual progress. Too often
people strive for dramatic progress, the swift and striking breakthrough everyone notices. Look at the claims of the popular starva-
tion diets: "lose 20 pounds in 20 days." Look at the advertisements
for exercise equipment, so confident in their power to change you
into a muscular—and well-greased—person in just 6 weeks. Right
before your eyes you can see the fat melt away, the muscles grow
and shine. This is the enticement of dramatic progress.

Such swift change, however, is usually gained at the cost of
great emotional and physical hardship. Gradual progress, which
involves no hardship, is the only route to your goals, but until this
chapter I didn't explain the process of making it recognizable—
what you should look for in your fitness program and how you
should hold onto it when you find it.

Collect your progress in a logbook; write a fitness autobiography. Fill it with your goals and the daily steps you take to reach them. Add graphs (see Figure 9.4) that plot your long-term progress in weight control, or in blood pressure reduction, or in strength and endurance, or in your yardstick flexibility rating. Highlight each milestone as you reach it. Don't look for dramatic progress; display your gradual progress dramatically.

Still, writing an autobiography isn't enough. You have to read it and then reread it—become so familiar with it that you know where to turn when you have a question about training, or when you want to give a friend advice based on personal experience, or when you just want a reason to smile. There will be plenty of those in your logbook.

Figure 9.4   *SEE THE BIG PICTURE*

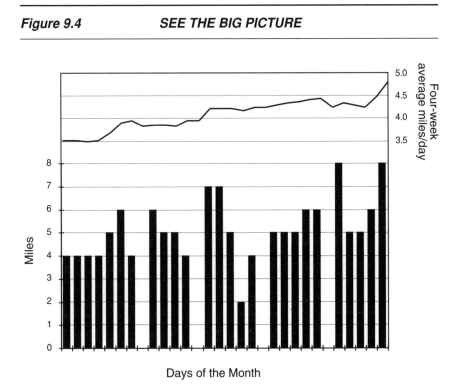

Days of the Month

A month's activity for a runner with the miles run each day (bar graph) and a four-week rolling average of miles per day (line graph) to show the trend.

• CHAPTER 10 •

PREVENTING INJURIES

When it comes to injuries, exercise has been given a bad rap. "Whenever I exercise, I get injured—I pull an Achilles tendon or hurt a knee," said an engineer in the Army Reserve. It's a common complaint, perhaps one echoed by you or someone you know. But injury is not an inevitable by-product of exercise. In fact sedentary people get injured far more often, losing twice as many workdays as exercisers and costing employers' health plans twice as much for illness and injury.

Unfortunately, Americans thirst for news, and bad news is what they usually get. Not long ago I stood at the starting line of a 10-K race and overheard the comment that so and so died while running this race several years ago. Sadly that incident did occur, but running by itself was not the villain. The heart attack victim had started his running program only six weeks before the race and wasn't conditioned well enough for such an exertion. But our long-term memory has a penchant, nurtured by the media, for remembering tragedy. Forgotten in the fine print are the details that led up to it. And no one gives any thought to what might have prevented it. All they remember is that so and so died while running.

Most people who have heart attacks have them while they are at rest, often while they sleep, and those who do have an attack during exercise are usually sedentary people who plunged themselves into an intense burst of activity more accurately described as self-abuse. Exercise is the opposite of self-abuse. When handled properly, it is the savior, not the killer, of people with health-risk factors or heart problems.

Steps You Can Take to Avoid Injuries

Once you commit yourself to an exercise program you usually become more interested in how your body works and how exercise can improve it. You already have the right attitude. What you need to know is how to avoid injuries, how to recognize them when they happen and what to do about them after that. This requires the knowledge I wish I had had when I started exercising. During my exercise career I've had three major injuries: two pulled muscles, one of the chest, the other of the shoulder, which pained me for months, and inflamed knees which plagued me for years. All these were avoidable. Let my bad experiences be the springboard to your good news.

Take a Stress Test

A first-line precaution is to take a stress test. If you have any of the health problems outlined in Chapter 1, ask your doctor about a stress test before you start an exercise program. A stress test will tell you if your heart has difficulty handling the extra work load and what your threshold of exercise intensity is, very important information because it enables you to exercise safely below that threshold. Some people with risk factors—for example, a family history of heart disease—may show normal results on a stress test. Interpret that to mean proceed with caution; intensify your workouts more gradually. You normally would increase the intensity of your workouts by no more than 10 percent every two weeks. If you have any risk factors, however, you would give yourself at least an extra week, increasing your exercise intensity every three or four weeks. This approach, well used by cardiac rehabilitation programs, strengthens the heart without any threat of overtaxing it. Safety is the first priority.

Warm Up Before Exercising

Another first-line caution often overlooked is to warm up before exercising. In our busy lives time is so scarce that we cut corners, eliminating any activities we consider unnecessary. Some activities are unnecessary, but warming-up isn't one of them. Warming-up prepares you for exercise, something that doesn't automatically happen when you step out of bed or walk around. As you warm up, you relax and focus on your workout; you gently push your heart to pump faster, you limber your joints with rotational movements, and stretch and activate your muscles. Altogether these muscle and joint changes make you much less vulnerable to pulls, tears, sprains, and the general impact of exercising. Yet many people refuse to use the 6 minutes it takes to do it.

Exercise Patience

The time factor is another common cause of injuries. Overflowing with enthusiasm, new exercisers tend to expand their workouts impatiently; they want to become fit now. But their bodies, needing time to recover and adjust, can't comply. Most people know that some progress comes from pushing yourself past the comfort zone, as in sprinting to become a faster runner. What they ignore is the second stage of the process: healing and recovery. This is exactly what leads to the overuse syndrome.

When you exercise beyond your normal intensity, you cause physiological and anatomical changes in bones, muscles, tendons, and ligaments. These changes are normal and healthy. But interrupt them with more exercise of the same intensity and you push yourself to the limit of your vulnerability. Bone, for example, responds to impact by reforming itself. While it reforms it is actually weaker, more vulnerable, and needs to be rested. If the bone is allowed to reform at rest, it will become stronger than before. If the bone's rest is interrupted by more high-impact activity while it's still reforming, it will break. This is how stress fractures happen. Muscles suffer a similar fate, tearing or becoming inflamed when they are not properly rested after unusual exertion. "Too much, too soon" doesn't make you tougher; it makes you weaker.

The Army realized this while training raw recruits into "lean, mean, fighting machines." In its eight-week basic training program, it had compressed more exercise and activities than many of the

recruits had ever done before. To adapt to this new level of activity, their bones and muscles began to reform. But the recruits were
never given a rest. Their weakened bones started to break, and their
muscles started to tear. The toll in stress fractures of the legs and
feet alone was so high that medicine was forced to overrule tradition with an order to drastically reduce impact activities during the
third week of basic training, about the time when most bone refor-
mation takes place.

Overuse injuries can be easily avoided if you comply with the
10 percent rule, which prohibits increasing amount, distance, duration (except when the original time is very short), or intensity by
more than 10 percent every two weeks. If you are running 10 miles
a week, don't increase it to 15—your body won't be prepared for it.
Nor will your body be prepared for an increase in running speed
from 10 minutes per mile to 8 minutes per mile, or the addition of
more than 10 percent of the poundage you use for weight lifting.

In these examples the 10 percent rule is easy to apply. Time,
speed, and weight are quite measurable. Intensity, however, isn't.
Exercise intensity is measured by your pulse rate. Some people may
find this method to be overly technical, a chore they don't want to
add to their workouts. If you feel this way, use the easy-day, hard-
day approach. On an easy day, do your regular workout; on a hard
day, increase the intensity. How much you increase the intensity and
how many hard workouts you do in a week depends on how you
feel. To prepare for race season a few years ago, I started running
intervals on Tuesdays and Thursdays. But by Sunday my legs still
hadn't recovered, so I cut back and ran intervals only once a week.

Well, that seems easy enough. All you have to do is know
when "too much" happens. But when will that be? Will you hear a
little voice in your ears telling you to slow down? Of course not.
That's why you record how you feel each day in an exercise logbook. Don't wait for that little voice to ring in your ears, and don't
trust your memory either. Today we all live in the fast lane; the days
blur together. "Was it yesterday or the day before when my legs felt
so tired?" you'll wonder, and your memory won't have the answer.

Recognize the Symptoms of Overtraining

Overuse that continues leads to overtraining. Commonly associated
with elite athletes, overtraining also happens to the amateur exer-

ciser, whose training program doesn't even come close to that of an Olympian. The amateur overtrainer is usually a competitive and disciplined person. He will insist on moving ahead too fast for his body to keep up and refuse to back off even when he reads the handwriting on his logbook. What complicates matters even more is that overtraining is so hard to recognize. It isn't an all-or-none, black-or-white phenomenon that strikes as soon as you go beyond a given work load. It sneaks up on you. And one person's overtraining symptoms won't be the same as another. Some overtrained people constantly feel tired, yet being true to the mind-set that drove them to overtrain and being unaware of what the problem really is, they respond to the fatigue and lackluster workouts with even more exercise. We all have bad days. But if bad days are the rule instead of the exception, it's time to take a closer look at yourself.

The following list contains the physical and emotional symptoms of overtraining. Of the emotional symptoms, the most telling one is that you don't enjoy your workouts any more and it's probably accompanied by other symptoms too.

Emotional symptoms

- Apathy toward or dread of workouts
- Apathy toward activities previously considered pleasurable
- Excessive tension, anxiety, or inability to relax
- Depressed mood
- Poor concentration

Physical symptoms

- Decreased exercise performance
- Inability to bounce back from intense workouts
- Increased muscle soreness or injuries
- More frequent illnesses
- Unexplained weight gain or weight loss
- Unexplained loose bowel movements or constipation
- Decreased appetite
- Morning heart rate (resting) 10 percent higher than usual

Alone, hard workouts may not be enough to cause overtraining. But when combined with other burdens, such as work or family crises, they can bring on the syndrome. If you have four or more symptoms, try cutting back on your workouts. Overtraining caught early disappears quickly; within two weeks you feel fresh again. More serious cases, however, that have gone on for months could take up to two months to correct.

Overtraining causes many people to give up exercise because they misinterpret their symptoms as a permanent condition, and this confusion is obvious when they try to explain why they quit. They'll tell you they got bored with exercise or just burned out. At a recent 10-K race I asked a bystander who used to run in all the local races why he wasn't at the starting line. His explanation was one of the most interesting descriptions of overtraining that I've heard. "I guess my body just ran out of miles," he said.

Use the Right Technique

Many people who don't overtrain get injured anyway. "How could I get injured when I wasn't even pushing myself?" they ask. The reason is not the duration or intensity of their workout, but their technique. By using good technique, you avoid injuries. Often exercisers sabotage it with their own enthusiasm or impatience, abruptly injuring themselves or slowly wearing down their muscles and joints until a full-blown injury develops.

Weight lifting, for example, requires that you lift weights slowly and smoothly through well-defined ranges of motion while maintaining the correct breathing pattern and posture. Yet many people jerk the weights, hold their breath, and slouch. Sit-ups are also victims of technical massacres. Instead of smoothly raising and lowering their torsos, people arch their backs and yank their heads. Cross-country skiing is an exercise that practically forces you to use a smooth motion, yet its technique, synchronized movements of arms and legs, feels awkward at first, and beginners fall to injury and frustration. But then most of us didn't grow up cross-country skiing; we grew up riding bikes. That must mean that cycling is a natural and therefore safe activity. Unfortunately it isn't—setting the wrong seat height can lead to injuries of the knees and back. Setting it too low keeps your knees bent at too small an angle throughout the peddling motion; setting it too high forces your knees to lock on the down peddle and puts an added strain on your back. During our years of pleasure riding, few of us gave much thought to our technique. Exercise riding demands more attention to that detail.

Running is another activity we grew up with, but as an exercise it's more than a pastime; it's a discipline that demands good technique, that your arms and legs move with a smooth rhythm, that your head be as still as possible, and that the twist of your torso be minimized while your arms swing by your waist in a forward and backward motion. If your stride is too long, your lead foot brakes you as it strikes the ground. If your stride is too short, you take more paces than necessary.

One common vein that runs through all exercise technique is that it be smooth and rhythmic. The body wasn't built to be jerked and jolted. During the start of a 10-K race I watched Julie Isphording, who was at that time a woman's Olympic marathon qualifier. She glided effortlessly and I noticed—as she pulled away from me—that her head wasn't bobbing like those of the runners around her. Observing professionals in your chosen sport is an excellent way to learn proper technique. Read the instruction booklets that come with your exercise equipment and the magazines that concentrate on your sport; they are full of expert advice and personal experience. Talk to longtime exercisers and trained professionals. Watch exercise programs and instruction videos. All around you there is information about exercise technique. Pay attention to it.

Equip Yourself Properly

Equally important is your equipment. To most exercisers this means machines—exercycles, rowing machines, weight-lifting machines—which should allow you to move smoothly through the motion at an even tension in the right directions. Not as obvious is another kind of equipment: what you wear. A runner, for example, must protect himself from the surface he runs on. The safest surface is a track. But tracks are inconvenient—one isn't on every block—and they are notoriously boring to run on. A grass surface, although kind on impact, is an uneven surface for feet to land on, exposing a runner to sprains. That leaves concrete and asphalt. These are the two hardest but most available running surfaces and good running technique alone will not protect you from the pounding your lower body will take; you also need good shoes.

Good shoes, an obvious accessory—but how many new exercisers know enough about them? In many sports—running, walking, cross-country skiing, tennis, basketball—your feet are the first point of impact. What harms your feet will also harm your ankles, knees, hips, and back. Some people might dismiss the importance of their feet; they row or cycle for exercise. But for anyone who spends time on their feet, even commuting or doing chores around the house, it is important to wear the right kind of shoes. When I began running, I wore an old pair of boat sneakers. I figured any sneakers were good for running. My knees told me they were not and a pair of well-cushioned running shoes relieved their pain. Now I wear running shoes whenever possible. A foot or knee problem doesn't have to happen during exercise.

Therefore, learn what foot type you have. One way to find out is to examine the wear on your shoes. But sometimes it's hard to make out a pattern of wear, especially when the shoes are well worn. Another way to identify your foot type is to use the footprint test: dampen the bottom of your foot and step onto a piece of paper. Although no two pair of feet look alike, your shoe wear or footprint will probably match one of the foot types in Figure 10.1.

The first category is "normal." Named to reflect its low vulnerability to injury, this kind of foot is also least likely to cause problems for the rest of your lower body—that is if you're in the 25 percent of the population lucky enough to have it. For a normal foot choose the most cushioned shoe.

The second category is the overpronating foot. Also called a "flat," "floppy," or "hypermobile" foot, an overpronating foot can develop inflammations of its connective tissue or tendons, and its excessive motion can lead to leg, knee, and hip injuries—bad news for the 50 percent of us who have it. If you are not a severe overpronator, wear motion-control shoes. If you are a severe overpronator, invest the time and money to have custom orthotics made, for only they can correct that much motion. Orthotics are shoe liners specifically designed to support and control your feet.

The last foot type is the supinator. A supinating foot, also called a "clunk," "rigid," or "high-arched" foot, doesn't need motion control. As one of its names suggest it's already too rigid, missing the motion necessary to spread the impact across the foot. Again, this will put your feet, legs, and knees at risk. Lessen the impact with well-cushioned shoes.

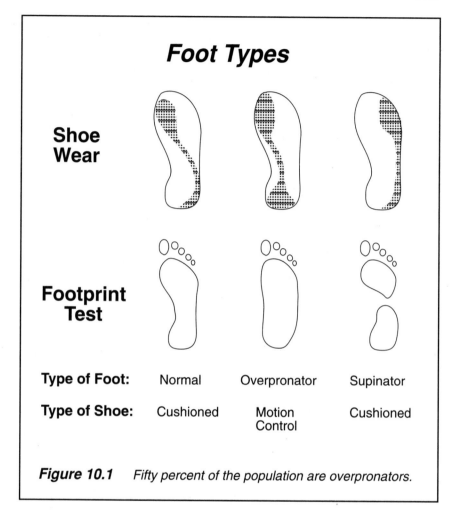

Foot Types

Shoe Wear

Footprint Test

Type of Foot:	Normal	Overpronator	Supinator
Type of Shoe:	Cushioned	Motion Control	Cushioned

Figure 10.1 Fifty percent of the population are overpronators.

I recommend motion-control shoes for overpronators only. That is not to say a normal or supinating foot would be harmed by such a shoe. But motion-control designs tend to have less cushioning, and there's no point in trading off your valuable cushioning for a feature you don't need.

Even to overpronators cushioning is sacred. That's why it's important to know that it won't last forever; cushioning begins to breakdown between 500 and 700 miles of wear. Shoes that have tread over 700 miles should be worn when you read the newspaper.

Aerobic exercise shoes have their own strict specifications for cushioning and motion control. They should be well cushioned in the forefoot (ball of foot), cupped in the rear for stability, and reinforced on the sides to prevent the foot from rolling inward and outward. In short, these shoes must offer protection. And in an injury-prone sport like aerobics, you need all the protection you can get.

Speaking of protection, do high-top sneakers offer more of it? A style frequently seen in basketball, high-tops, it might seem, can prevent ankle and foot injuries. They don't. High-tops are a fashion feature only. What you see is all you get.

Whenever you buy exercise shoes, know what you need before you walk into a store. Then, wearing *both* shoes, walk on an uncarpeted surface. Remember, you're not looking for well-advertised shoes, or expensive shoes, or pretty shoes; you are looking for shoes that are right for your feet. If they are not comfortable, don't buy them. (See Figure 10.2 for a checklist of steps you can take to avoid injuries.)

ARE YOUR ACHES AND PAINS NORMAL OR ARE YOU INJURED?

There is no such equation as pain equals injury. Often your muscles will feel sore after a new or intensified exercise. But this is not an injury; it's a normal sign that you have overloaded those muscles and that they are conditioning themselves in response to it. Beyond the discomfort are fitter muscles.

"That's good to know," you may say, "but what can I do about the pain?" You have two approaches. If you are absolutely sure that you'll be sore after a workout, follow it with 400 milligrams of ibuprofen and repeat the dose every 6 hours for the next 24 hours. But don't take this as a prescription to treat phantom pain. Every workout won't cause muscle pain afterward. If you're not sure whether you'll be sore, wait. Then if pain does develop, take the same doses of ibuprofen for the next 24 hours.

So much for the normal aches and pains of exercise. But how do you differentiate them from an injury? Many exercisers can't unless they have an obvious mishap where they fall and twist a knee or an ankle or they feel the sudden and searing pain of a severe muscle pull. Without such a disaster they assume the sore

Figure 10.2	**PRECAUTIONS CHECKLIST**
☐ **Stress Test**	If you have any health problems, ask your doctor about a stress test. Will tell you if your heart has difficulty handling the extra work load of exercise. Indicates maximum safe exercise intensity.
☐ **Warm Up**	Take the time to warm up properly with these four steps: 1. Light aerobic exercise to give your heart a wake-up call. 2. Rotational movements for your joints — head to ankles. 3. Performance stretching — all areas of your body. 4. Very slowly begin your chosen exercise.
☐ **Patience**	Follow the "10 percent" rule: don't increase the amount, distance, duration or intensity of your workout by more than 10 percent every two weeks. Don't exercise hard two days in a row; alternate workouts with the easy day, hard day approach.
☐ **Over-training**	Recognize symptoms of overtraining such as • Decreased performance • Apathetic attitude • Increased soreness • Excessive tension • Frequent illness • Depressed mood • Decreased appetite • Poor concentration and cut back on your workout.
☐ **Technique**	Maintain smooth, natural motions. Seek a comfortable rhythm. Observe professionals or elite athletes in your chosen activity.
☐ **Equipment**	Make sure equipment matches your purpose and has smooth-acting mechanisms, uniform tension or speed, and stable construction. Wear running shoes to suit your foot type and replenish them frequently.

knee or ankle or calf muscle is a passing vestige of a workout. What they don't realize is that some injuries develop slowly, festering over weeks, or in the case of certain stress fractures, months. Stress fractures are small cracks in the bone, usually in the leg or foot, caused by the cumulative effects of impact. Other slow-developing injuries are not so obvious. One is tendonitis, an inflammation of the tissue that connects muscles to bones. Another is cartilage breakdown. Where the bones touch, they are covered by a flexible, slick layer called cartilage, which wears down or breaks from abnormal impact. As with stress fractures, cartilage and tendon injuries plague the legs and feet, but they also frequently occur in many other areas of the body.

These slow-developing injuries result from the cumulative stresses from a mechanical problem with the body. Perhaps a joint can't move properly. Or the joint can move properly, but the activity you are subjecting it to forces it into an unnatural motion. Consider the runner who runs on one side of a banked road, and then crosses over to the other side and runs back. It's a safe route: he is always facing traffic, and he can see what's happening on the road ahead. What he can't see is what's happening to his knees, hips, and back. Continually pounded on a tilted running surface, they get excessively stressed.

For many slow-developing injuries, the ultimate cure is not a prescription, or physical therapy, or surgery—although those may be needed to repair the damage. Back to the runner on the banked road. If the runner ran up and down one side of the road, the extra stress of a tilted road would be shared by both sides of his body, thus decreasing its effect. Or he could get rid of the extra stress altogether by running on a flat surface.

An excellent example of a nonmedical cure is my overcoming a chronic knee inflammation. For years knee pain and swelling kept me from running—and at times forced me to walk with a pronounced limp. An arsenal of anti-inflammatories didn't help, and neither did knee surgery. My running career was over. With that depressing realization, I began looking for an exercise that would give me a good aerobic workout without pounding my knees. The exercise I found was cross-country skiing. It felt great to exercise regularly again, and as I skied on my machine, strengthening my quadriceps with every stroke, a surprising thing happened: my knee problems disappeared.

Years of chronic knee problems and their eventual cure taught me a valuable lesson: all the drugs, surgery, and knee braces in the world weren't going to cure me. I had to strengthen my quadriceps and cut down on my running mileage.

My knee problems were the perfect example of a slow-developing injury. Other injuries happen suddenly and are easily recognized; the pain, swelling, and redness cannot be misinterpreted as delayed muscle soreness. Three kinds of injuries fall into this category: sprains, strains, and bruises. Typically, a sprain is an over-stretched ligament, a strain is an overstretched or torn muscle or tendon, and a bruise is a bleeding muscle. If you have any of these, you know you are injured.

WHAT TO DO IF YOU GET INJURED

To a dedicated exerciser, an injury is a supreme insult. "Why did this happen to me?" is the standard reaction and the emotional turmoil quickly equals the injury's physical discomfort. But this is not the time to brood. Take immediate action by applying ice to the injured area for 20 minutes, and then for the next 48 hours continue icing it every hour when possible, while keeping it elevated and applying constant compression (don't impair circulation). Commonly referred to as the RICE approach—Rest, Ice, Compression, Elevation (see Figure 10.3)—this treatment should not preclude the use of moist heat later in the healing process. Moist heat works well during a reintroduction to exercise. Applied for 10 minutes before each

Figure 10.3	INJURY TREATMENT
RICE	Use the RICE approach — Rest, Ice, Compression, Elevation. Ice for 20 minutes whenever possible over 48-hour period. Never allow ice to contact the skin directly; place a thin cloth between the ice and the skin. Ice should also be applied after workouts as the injury heals. Don't impair circulation with compression. The limb must be elevated above the heart.
Medication	Take a short course (5 - 7 days) of over-the-counter naproxen, ibuprofen, or aspirin — every 4 to 6 hours for ibuprofen or aspirin, twice a day for naproxen. Do NOT miss doses.
Moist Heat	Apply moist heat to the injured area after swelling has receded. Apply before exercising or stretching.
Stretch	Stretch the injured area to eliminate inflammation from tendons and connective tissue and to induce proper healing. Don't stretch to point of pain.

workout, it increases blood flow to the injured area, thereby preparing it to be mobilized again. Bear in mind that this advice is for minor injuries. If the pain and swelling are serious or persist beyond one week, see a doctor. A doctor can X-ray the area to determine if there is a fracture, and if necessary, immobilize it with a device designed just for that purpose.

Visiting the Doctor

If you do have to see a doctor, do so with the right attitude. As a resident at New York's Bellevue hospital, I had a patient with uncontrollable high blood pressure. John Doe, as I'll call him, had been told to drastically cut back the salt in his diet, yet he continued to eat anything he wanted to, including hot dogs for breakfast. One day while looking over his chart, I decided I had to change his medication; the one he was on wasn't counteracting the effect of his incredibly salty diet. Maybe another medication could do a better job. But when I told Mr. Doe about the change, he became exasperated and shouted, "How am I supposed to get better if you guys keep changing the medications on me?"

Many patients feel as Mr. Doe did—that the doctor is solely responsible for their recovery, while they passively sit back and watch. But this attitude is self-destructive. Bystanders feel helpless and angry. Participants feel as if they are helping to heal their injury, an attitude that keeps them positive and focused on resuming their fitness program. By taking an active role in your recovery, you give control to the person who is in the position to do the most good—yourself.

But you can't participate if you don't know what to do; you need information. That's where your doctor comes in. Besides diagnosing and prescribing, your doctor should also be answering questions. Implied here is that you ask questions. Doctors are not mind readers. Nor will they try to answer every question you might have. It's your responsibility to ask them.

Obviously it's not enough to know that you should ask questions; it's not even enough to know what questions to ask. You must remember to ask them. So often the anxiety of the moment blots out any questions you may have about the injury, about the prescription, about the surgery. Then the visit is over and the questions start popping up. This is the rule, not the exception.

Your job as the involved patient is to make it the exception by writing down your questions before the visit (see Figure 10.4). If other questions occur to you while your doctor is answering one on your list—and they will—just ask him or her to stop, while you write them down. In fact, write down the answers to all your questions as well. Writing down the answers helps you not only to remember the answers, but to listen to them in the first place. Most patients don't fully listen to what their doctor is saying; they're too busy wondering who'll watch the kids or how many days they'll miss work. They miss what is probably the information most important to them.

Figure 10.4   ***QUESTIONS FOR YOUR DOCTOR***

Injury   What caused my injury?
               How and when should I stretch to restore range of motion?
               Will I feel pain as I heal? How should I respond to pain?
               Will seeing a physical therapist help?
               How rapidly should my recovery progress?
               What can I do to prevent a recurrence?
               Should I strengthen certain muscle groups?
               What alternative exercises can I safely do?

Surgery   What are the dangers with this operation?
               What are the chances it will cure the problem?
               Can surgery make it worse?
               How much total rest and rehabilitation is required?

Medication * Is this medication the gentlest possible on my stomach?
               Are there other common side effects I should know about?
               What can I do to decrease side effects?
               Are there other medications I should avoid while taking this one?
               Will this medication also serve as a pain killer?

               * *Anti-inflammatory medications.*

Medications

Whether you see a doctor or not, a short course of anti-inflammatory medication immediately following the injury will ease the symptoms for a time. Of the over-the-counter anti-inflammatories, aspirin is the most common and least toxic. Next comes ibuprofen, more effective than aspirin when taken in 400- or 600-milligram doses, and for a while considered to be *the* nonprescription medication for injuries. Then naproxen entered the market. Formerly available as a prescription only, naproxen is the most effective anti-inflammatory and it is taken only twice a day. The less frequent doses make it easier to take with meals, cutting down on the possibility of stomach irritation. But even more important is that it's easier to remember two doses than it is to remember four. How many times have you forgotten to take a medication?

After naproxen, you graduate to prescription medications. In general, prescription anti-inflammatories are more effective than over-the-counter, but these results are had for a price: expense and side effects. The most common side effects are stomach and gastrointestinal problems. If you can avoid these—the best way is to religiously take the medication with enough food—you can get dramatic relief.

But don't expect miracles from these or any other medications. If you want a medication to work, you have to take it regularly. Taking doses haphazardly, as many people tend to do, delays or nullifies a medication's therapeutic effect. Even worse is when a patient stops taking a medication before they are supposed to. "It wasn't working," they complain. They expected it to squash the pain, swelling, and redness in a few days, when the process really takes at least a week, maybe two.

This discussion assumes that you have no allergies to or a history of side effects from other over-the-counter drugs or prescription anti-inflammatories. If you've had a reaction to any over-the-counter medication, consult a doctor before taking an over-the-counter anti-inflammatory. If your doctor is prescribing one, make sure he or she knows about any past reactions you've had to medications.

One group of medications that you'll never need to use are the sports rubs and creams. Why? Because they don't work. Except for one expensive prescription cream containing capsaicin (not capsaicin oleoresin), these products don't even decrease the pain, let alone the inflammation. Instead what they do is *mask* the pain. By causing a mild irritation of the skin, they deflect your attention from the sore joint or muscle. Doctors call these counter-irritants. You should call them a waste of money. They do little more than get on your clothing.

MANAGING INJURIES WITH EXERCISE

Following an injury calmly reexamine your program. Perhaps you recently expanded or intensified your exercise routine, or perhaps you're going through a career or family crisis—any number of factors could have combined to cause it.

Many injuries are caused by overuse (see Figure 10.5), and the best prescription for them is to cross-train with an exercise that doesn't put as much emphasis on the overused muscles. Such a regimen should also strengthen neglected muscles. Frequently, overuse injuries also point to a muscle imbalance, where a set of overused muscles is much stronger than a set of underused ones. Exercise programs, for example, that overwork the quadriceps with excessive biking, stairclimbing, or hill running typically neglect the hamstrings. Strong quadriceps and weak hamstrings is a common muscle imbalance that frequently leads to injury. Cause a sudden, strong contraction of the quadriceps—running abruptly or dashing upstairs—and the weaker hamstrings, unable to withstand the force, get overstretched or torn. By cross-training with an exercise that strengthens the hamstrings, such as biking with toe clips (the upstroke exercises the hamstrings), you can avoid a muscle imbalance while adding to your aerobic workout.

In the preceding paragraph, I discuss cross-training as an aerobic option. But a cross-training exercise can also be anaerobic. If you have a weak muscle group, weight lifting, which is much more muscle specific than aerobic exercise, can isolate and strengthen it efficiently. The weak hamstrings could be corrected with reverse leg lifts.

Always look to your cross-training if an injury prevents you from doing your primary exercise. When my bunion flared, I could not push off the victimized toe, and therefore had to stop my running speedwork. But my fitness program didn't suffer. I was able to replace the speedwork with stairclimbing because my stairclimber

Figure 10.5	*DIAGNOSING INJURIES*		
Injury	**Symptoms**	**Causes**	**Avoidance**
Muscles			
Hamstrings Quadriceps Groin Neck/Shoulder Back Calf	Pain that decreases somewhat as you warm up, swelling, redness, warmth.	Muscle imbalance, sudden powerful contraction of opposing muscle group, overtraining, overuse, inflexibility, previous injury, trauma.	Strengthen muscle, warm up, cut back, cross-train, performance stretching, developmental stretching.
Tendons			
Elbow Knee Foot Shoulder Leg Hand	Pain decreases somewhat as you warm up then returns when you stop, swelling, redness, warmth.	Sudden powerful contraction of muscle attached to tendon, overtraining, overuse, inflexibility, previous injury.	Follow the 10 percent rule, developmental stretching.
Bones			
Foot Leg (shin) Thigh	Pain gets worse as you exercise.	Overtraining, overuse (for high impact exercise), trauma.	Follow the 10 percent rule, cross-train with low impact exercise, adequate calcium intake.
Joints (ligaments & cartilage)			
Ankle Knee Foot Elbow/Shoulder Hip Back	Pain gets worse as you exercise.	Overtraining, overuse, trauma, mechanical vulnerability, muscle imbalance.	Follow the 10 percent rule, strengthen supportive muscle groups, avoid wraps or braces unless prescribed.

allowed me to stand with my toes hanging off the front of the pedal, leaving my bunion in peace.

In some cases the alternate exercise can even be therapeutic. People suffering from inflammations of the Achilles tendon or the connective tissue along the bottom of the feet can safely bicycle or cross-country ski. But if they cross-country ski, they get the added benefit of a foot-stretching motion that promotes healing.

The point is that injuries don't have to stop you from exercising. If you can't do one exercise, try another—there will always be an alternate exercise you can do. You just have to look for it. And don't rely solely on your doctor as a source of advice. For my chronically injured knees I kept getting the same advice from doctors: bicycle or swim. Today my knees are stronger and healthier than ever, yet cycling still bothers them on occasion, and as for swimming, the leg kicking made my knees grind and ache—definitely not what you want from a rehabilitory exercise. Doctors must deal with averages. They will recommend what works for most patients with a given injury, and they are right to do so.

Many patients, however, fall outside the realm of average. Always gather as much information as you can from physical therapists, from personal trainers, from other exercisers, from books and magazines. What finally saved my knees was the improbable exercise of cross-country skiing—improbable because it was a weight bearing exercise, and the averages decreed that my injury was worsened by the burden of weight. The physical therapist who first put me on a cross-country ski machine said, "You're the first patient to ever use one of these machines." I don't mind being a guinea pig when the experiment ends up such a blazing success.

Some injuries may require part of your body to be immobilized. In that case there is an important prelude to exercise: regaining your range of motion. Often this is as hard as getting over the injury itself. The body was not meant to be immobilized. Immobilize it only if a doctor says you should. Then start moving it again as soon as possible.

If you get an injury, don't let it divorce you from the exercise your mind and body need; use it instead as an opportunity to learn. See Figure 10.6 for exercises that will help you overcome common injuries. Review it with an open mind and positive attitude. Who knows, you may discover an exercise that you'll enjoy for the rest of your life.

Figure 10.6　　　　　　**INJURY MANAGEMENT**

Injury	Causes	Treatment	Discontinue Excercises
Shoulder	Imbalance of opposing muscle Overtraining Overuse Trauma	RICE Moist heat (after swelling gone) Anti-inflammatories	Rowing CC skiing w/ upper body Swimming Aerobics
Upper Back	Imbalance of opposing muscle Overtraining Overuse Trauma	RICE Moist heat (after swelling gone) Anti-inflammatories	CC skiing w/ upper body Rowing Swimming Aerobics
Lower Back	Weak abdominals Lower body inflexibility Overtraining Overuse	RICE Moist heat (after swelling gone) Anti-inflammatories Relaxation exercises	Running Rowing Aerobics CC skiing w/ upper body
Hamstrings	Imbalance of opposing muscle Overtraining Overuse Inflexibility	RICE Moist heat (after swelling gone) Anti-inflammatories Stretch	Running Rowing CC skiing Aerobics
Knee	Overuse, Trauma Mechanical vulnerability Sudden contraction of muscle / tendon	RICE Anti-inflammatories	Running Aerobics
Ankle	Excessive flexibility Overuse Trauma	RICE Anti-inflammatories	Running Aerobics CC skiing Stairclimbing
Achilles	Sudden contraction of muscle / tendon Worn / wrong shoes Overuse Inflexibility	RICE Anti-inflammatories Shoes for overpronating Stretch	Running (fast) Hill running
Shin Splints	Overtraining Overuse Muscle imbalance Inflexibility	RICE Anti-inflammatories	Running Aerobics

Figure 10.6 (continued).

Recovery Exercises	Prevention Exercises	
Running / walking CC skiing w/o upper body Cycling Stairclimbing	Lat pulldowns Upright rowing Bench press	 Lat pulldown Upright rowing
CC skiing w/o upper body Cycling Stairclimbing	Reverse flies One-arm rowing Lat pulldowns	 Reverse flies One-arm rowing
CC skiing w/o upper body Cycling Stairclimbing Swimming	Sit-ups Reverse leg lifts Back raises Hamstring curls Hamstring stretch	 Reverse leg lift
Cycling Stairclimbing Swimming	Hamstring kickbacks Hamstring curls Reverse leg lifts	 Hamstring kickback Hamstring curl
CC skiing Cycling Stairclimbing Rowing Swimming	Leg extensions Straight leg lifts Hamstring curls	 Leg extension Straight leg lift
Cycling (ankle stabilized) Swimming Water running	Foot spreader Toe walking Heel walking	Foot spreader *(Bind feet and spread them apart at the toes)*
CC skiing Cycling Rowing Swimming	Toe raises Wall squat	 Toe raises Wall squat
CC skiing Cycling Rowing	Foot raises	Foot raises

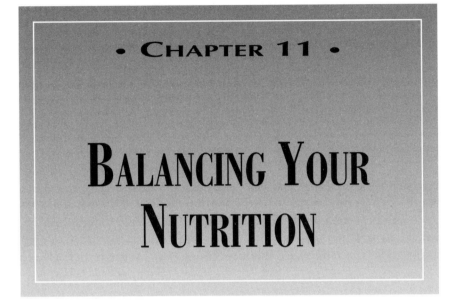

· CHAPTER 11 ·

BALANCING YOUR NUTRITION

Marvin and Dullus lived disciplined lives. They exercised regularly and ate a balanced, low-fat diet. No wonder they were slim and healthy. Then something happened, and they started to eat more and more, gorging themselves into a state of grotesque obesity. Scientists studying Marvin and Dullus' gluttony were not surprised; in fact, they had caused it. Marvin and Dullus were laboratory rats.

What had pushed them over the edge, into a quagmire of uncontrollable eating? The answer is a change in their diets. Fed regular rat chow, Marvin and Dullus thrived without overeating. But when scientists switched them to a sweetened, high-fat diet—aptly called the Supermarket Diet—they gorged themselves continually. Executives have something in common with Marvin and Dullus: the Supermarket Diet, an addictive combination of cakes, cookies, fried foods, crunchy snacks, and creamy desserts. Sweet, fatty foods that make you crave more sweet, fatty foods.

Yet this is the average American diet, and it serves you an irony. Fat and sugar, nutrients that seem to stand for energy, actually sap you of it, saddling you with extra pounds and corroding the cardiovascular system you work so hard to keep healthy. In short, the average American diet isn't for exercisers—it's not even for the average American rat.

Almost everyone claims to know something about proper nutrition, but few people consistently practice it. Most people, including executives, have poor nutritional habits because, until recently these habits were considered healthy. For example, in the 1960s, the diet with the most protein was thought to be the healthiest, most energy-producing one. Protein was revered even though large dollops of fat came with it. Back then fat was not declared a nutritional outlaw; cholesterol was. And cholesterol shared the most unwanted list with sugars and starches, the famous carbohydrate bandits. Their crime—they made you fat.

Nutrition headlines are different today. Yet generations of adults are still burdened with solidly ingrained eating habits forged in decades past, and these habits will not easily release their grip.

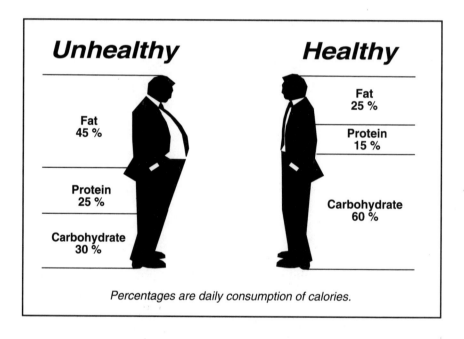

Percentages are daily consumption of calories.

FAT IS A CLOAKED TAKEOVER ARTIST
AND RUTHLESS COMPETITOR

Today, fats make up between 40 and 50 percent of the calories in diets of most Americans. Even for a slim person this is too much. The U.S. Dietary Guidelines, which suggest that 30 percent of your calories come from fat, is still too lax. Better advice comes from the private sector's, researchers at hospitals and universities. Basing their standards on the outcome of epidemiological studies, these authorities issued more stringent limits: of total calories, fat should make up only 25 percent, with saturated fat below 10 percent. For many people this means cutting their fat intake in half.

But some fat is necessary and useful in the diet. It is an indispensable component of cellular structure, and it aids metabolism by promoting the absorption of certain vitamins. Fat, however, is most noted for, or better said notorious as, a lightweight form of energy storage. Housed in the adipose tissue, fat's role in our existence has changed over time. During the early evolution of humankind, it was needed just to survive. Today we work hard—even pay others—to get rid of it.

Fats are labeled by their degree of saturation: saturated, unsaturated or polyunsaturated, and most recently monounsaturated. With the exception of monounsaturates, the more saturated a fat is, the more dangerous to your health it is, a detail that steers us away from animal fats because they are saturated and towards vegetable fats because they are unsaturated. A fat's melting point reveals how saturated it is. Highly saturated beef fat is solid at room temperature, and vegetable oils, which are high in unsaturates, are liquid at room temperature.

Unfortunately, a process called hydrogenation clouds the melting point test. Hydrogenation makes vegetable oils solid at room temperature, so they can exist as a stick of margarine or as a solid shortening. But this process also strips these oils of their innocence.

After hydrogenation, the newly solid vegetable oils contain substances called trans fatty acids, which increase the cholesterol levels in the blood. Technically these solid vegetable oils are not saturated. Your body, however, says they are. Up goes your cholesterol when it was supposed to go down. So much for guarding yourself against cardiovascular disease—or breast or colon cancer, two other diseases linked to fat.

The government is helping to expose fat hidden in packaged foods. Recent regulations have made label reading, which was a tricky if not impossible task, much easier. But the regulations are silent for a multitude of fresh dairy and meat products. Hence, you have to be a determined detective to uncover the fat in your diet. To compound the problem, fat is more than twice as dense in calories as the other nutrients, making it doubly lethal in adding pounds to your torso. If you don't get anything else out of this chapter on nutrition, get it into your mind that fat is your enemy.

OVERRATED PROTEIN HAS AN ALLIANCE WITH FAT

But executives do not live on fat alone. Protein is also well loved. In fact, it has a mystique about it: it's good for you and it grows muscles. Males, in particular, believe that protein has some magical strength-inducing, performance-enhancing power. These beliefs, together with tradition, lead them to eat twice as much protein as they need.

How much protein you need depends on your weight. For every 2.2 pounds you need to consume 0.7 grams of protein a day. If you weigh 150 pounds, for example, eating 50 grams of protein daily will cover all your body's needs. But this estimate is for sedentary people and no one should be sedentary. For those who do aerobic exercise regularly, endurance train, or weight lift to build muscle (as opposed to maintaining it), the estimate must be increased to 1 gram of protein per 2.2 pounds, or 70 grams of protein a day for a 150-pound person. In calories, it works out to about 15 percent of the total consumed. Now that's probably much less protein than you've been eating, but it more accurately reflects your needs than your habits do.

Proteins are made up of amino acids, some which your body can construct (nonessential) and some which you must eat (essential). What makes a food a high-quality or complete protein is that it contains all the essential amino acids. Beef, pork, poultry, fish, and dairy products qualify as complete proteins. But look at the fat contents of milk, cheese, red meats, and dark meat poultry; it's high enough to saturate your diet with fat.

In general, plant proteins contain less fat, but they are incomplete, lacking in some of the essential amino acids, and must be supplemented with other proteins. It's a mix-and-match process. For example, a small amount of complete cheese protein mixed with a large amount of incomplete pasta protein yields a large amount of protein that is as high in quality as the cheese alone. Still, cheese is a complete protein. Can you combine two incompletes to get a complete? The answer is yes: by combining pasta with lentils or any legumes, you create a complete protein. Pasta isn't the only versatile incomplete protein around. Rice and bread also lend themselves to combinations that yield high-quality proteins.

Protein's most famous and confusing function is as a building block of muscles, a fact that leads many people to believe that, by eating protein, they will develop muscles. Not true. Protein *helps* to build muscles when you exercise. Otherwise, it is a material used for repairing muscles worn or injured by normal daily activities. Besides construction work, proteins also make up enzymes, drivers of chemical reactions in the body.

Some diets claim that the body excretes excess protein. This is an unhealthy fallacy. When you eat too much protein, more than your body needs for repairs and enzymes, your body breaks down the excess, excreting *one part of it* in the urine and storing the rest of it on your waist and hips as fat. Nowadays no one needs the fat that excess protein lays on them.

CARBOHYDRATES ARE THE "WHITE KNIGHTS"

Carbohydrates are finally getting the respect they deserve. Long crowded out of the diet by fats and proteins, carbohydrates are now considered our body's most important energy source. Most executives need to double their carbohydrate intake from about 30 percent of their total calories to 60 percent. Drastic as this may seem, it is a must. Too few carbohydrates in your diet throws off the entire nutritional balance of your body.

Here's an analogy of what happens. Suppose you are stranded on the tundra with a small "protein" wood supply. Do you burn it for heat or use it to build a shelter? If you burn it for heat, you'll have no shelter. Such is the fate of your lean body mass, mostly protein, when you don't eat enough carbohydrates; in desperation the body breaks down its protein and burns it for energy. To survive on the tundra, you need "protein" wood and "carbohydrate" coal. Coal will burn longer and hotter than wood. Then, with a reliable heat source, you are free to build a shelter with your "protein" wood.

But not all carbohydrates are created equal; some feed your muscles better than others. There are two kinds of carbohydrates: simple and complex. Complex carbohydrates come from plants that store energy as starch, such as wheat and potatoes. The body breaks down these carbohydrates through a long and complicated process to yield the sugar, glucose—the true food of muscles. During processing it is gradually released into the bloodstream. Simple carbohydrates are already sugars, so they need minimal processing to become available to the muscles. Therefore, simple carbohydrates would seem to be a tasty, efficient way to feed your muscles—and they would be, were it not for a hormone called insulin.

When the bloodstream gets a large rush of sugar, as it does when you eat sugar, your body responds with a large surge of insulin. Insulin promotes the uptake of sugar by the cells. But these aren't muscle cells being loaded; they are fat cells. By sweeping the sugar into your fat cells, insulin actually decreases the carbohydrate sugar available to your muscle cells. It's house cleaning gone awry. Insulin cleans the blood of sugar and locks it in adipose tissue where you don't want it. A candy bar snack before a workout worsens this scenario. Not only does insulin deny your muscles the candy bar's sugar; it also *locks* normally available fat energy inside your fat cells, because the process of moving sugar into the fat cells temporarily prevents any outflow. Now your muscles are deprived of a second energy source.

Besides the insulin reaction, simple sugars cause other problems. They usually bring along fat, flooding you with many calories, but no vitamins or fiber. Even worse, they are condensed into small packages. How long does it take to eat a cupcake or candy bar? Perhaps you should have another one—or two. Obviously the eating pleasure is fleeting. As for the hunger that drove you to eat the first candy bar, that remains unsatisfied. You want more. Numerous theories try to explain this drive to eat more; some of them indict insulin. Whatever the reason, learn the lesson Marvin and Dullus, the fat laboratory rats, taught. Don't eat sugary foods often.

But do eat complex carbohydrates often. This is especially relevant to exercisers because complex carbohydrates are "exerciser friendly." Frequent exercise teaches muscles to prepare for more exercise; hence they plan for future energy needs by seizing and storing excess carbohydrates. The muscles of sedentary people don't need to plan. Always inactive, these muscles have no need for extra energy, and they allow excess carbohydrates to slide into the fat tissue—just one of the reasons sedentary people get fat.

Don't misinterpret the sedentary muscles' disinterest in extra carbohydrates as a sign that they already have enough energy. On the contrary, they lack energy, and they afflict you with a feeling of tiredness, an endless lethargy. As a regular exerciser, you'll feel more energetic, your muscles always primed with carbohydrates and ready for action.

GOOD AND BAD CHOLESTEROL

Cholesterol is not a protein, fat, or carbohydrate. It is a cyclic alcohol, a substance that for years reigned as king of the dark side of our diets, though it has recently been dethroned by saturated fats. Still, cholesterol remains a substance to avoid.

Yet we can't live without it. Cholesterol is part of every cell membrane, of every digestive process, of every steroid hormone in our body. But because it is produced by the liver, we don't need to ingest it with our food; hence we have been pounded with warnings not to eat cholesterols that too much of it in the long run will kill us.

A waxy substance, cholesterol is insoluble in blood, and has to travel around the circulatory system in a vehicle. The technical term for this vehicle is lipoprotein. It operates much like a taxi on the streets of a large city, picking up fares and dropping them off. But cholesterol doesn't ride alone; it has a favorite riding companion called triglycerides (a component of fat). Some taxis carry more cholesterol than triglycerides. Some carry more triglycerides than cholesterol. If a taxi is carrying more triglycerides, it is less dense and lighter, earning it the name low-density lipoprotein or LDL. When too many LDL taxis cruise around, a traffic jam develops and small portions of them oxidize, damaging artery walls and dropping off cholesterol, which eventually chokes off blood flow. Call the police. Better yet, call another taxi and densely pack it with cholesterol to form a high-density lipoprotein (HDL). Though this taxi also contains cholesterol, it does no harm; it simply takes the cholesterol back to the liver where it can stay out of trouble.

Saturated fats are a major concern because they actually have a bigger effect on cholesterol levels than cholesterol itself. The more saturated fats in a diet, the higher the LDL level is, and as it rises so does the probability of developing atherosclerosis. But this condition can be reversed if you eat less saturated fat. Not only will this reduce LDL and increase HDL; it will heal some of the damage done to the arteries. The great thoroughfares remain open.

HDL's role in this drama obsoletes the simple "cholesterol level" as a gauge of heart health. What you need to know are your levels of HDL, LDL, and VLDL (very-low-density lipoprotein). True, high readings for LDL and VLDL mean trouble, but the ratio of total cholesterol to HDL is more accurate (see Figure 11.1). Worry if you have a ratio over 4.5. Proceed with caution if you have one between 4.5 and 3.5. And be proud if your ratio is under 3.5—your future looks bright.

VITAMINS, MINERALS, AND FLUIDS

It's not hard to understand why vitamins have received so much publicity lately if you pay attention to the latest research findings. Researchers are busily looking for cures and preventions of diseases, for boosters of energy and strength, even for ways to retard

Figure 11.1	CHOLESTEROL AND HDL RATIOS	
Total Cholesterol	**HDL Ratio**	**Remedial Action**
Under 175	N/A	Usually good unless there is a very low proportion of HDL. Treat with diet.
Over 175	Over 4.5	Treat with diet.
Over 200	3.5 to 4.5	Treat with diet.
Over 250	Over 3.5	Medication if diet doesn't produce satisfactory results.
Over 300	Below 3.5	Try diet first.
Over 300	Over 3.5	Medication and diet.

aging, through what must be the most direct and, of course, easiest route—putting a pill in your mouth. So demand signals and supply answers. Onto the market marches an army of supplements that can turn a careless diet into a prototype of nutritional perfection. Food manufacturers also hear the call. Vitamins lost during the processing of food are added back; in fact vitamins never present in the food are thrown in. Into fruit punch goes calcium. Into milk goes vitamin D. Into cereal goes an array of B vitamins, along with a nice helping of vitamins A and C. The cereal names alone—Special K, Total, King Vitamin—will tell the story. But the followers of this king have only a vague idea of what vitamins do. When asked why she took vitamins, the president of a local Chamber of Commerce replied, "They cleanse my body."

It's time you start with a cleansed slate. Vitamins help the body use proteins, carbohydrates, and fats efficiently. After food is eaten, the body must quickly break it down into useful building blocks with the chemical reactions of digestion and absorption. To accelerate these reactions, it uses enzymes. Vitamins are the helpers of enzymes.

An enzyme is like a washing machine. Load it with fat, protein, and carbohydrate clothing, add vitamin detergent, and it turns on.

The result: clean clothing that is more useful to the body and a washing machine, unchanged, awaiting its next wash. If the washing machine could have washed the clothes without detergent, it would do an incomplete job. Add detergent and the clothing comes out clean. But don't add too much. This detergent is concentrated; only small amounts are needed for each wash.

This doesn't tell you exactly how much vitamins you need. Unfortunately, even experts struggle with the question, and when asked, they respond with endless combinations of servings of leafy green vegetables and whole grain products. But man does not live on broccoli and whole wheat bread alone. Nor does he have the time to figure out which vitamins are lacking in his diet. Therefore let's generalize. It's unlikely that an executive suffers from severe deficiencies—if anything, what you need to cover is the chance that you are not getting enough of certain vitamins and minerals, a low-grade deficiency. For that all you need is a high-potency multivitamin. It's the most economical health insurance you can buy.

A good supplement should supply 100 to 150 percent of all the vitamins and minerals for which USRDAs have been set except biotin, magnesium, calcium, iron, and phosphorous. It should also dissolve quickly so the body can absorb its contents and have an expiration date that clearly shows the year and month it expires. If a supplement doesn't have an expiration date, don't buy it.

By taking vitamin supplements (see Figure 11.2) you shore up your nutritional foundation. But don't take too much. Remember, the washing machine needs very little detergent. If you saturate your wash with it, the machine will malfunction, and the clothing will come out soapy. In short, your health will be impaired. Too much of a good thing is harmful. It's tempting, however, to think otherwise when you hear or read about new wives' tales; how more energy and improved athletic performance are yours for just taking more B vitamins. What could be easier? Certainly not the truth. These theories are not supported by research.

Figure 11.2   VITAMINS AND MINERALS

Vit. / Min.	USRDA	Source	Function
A *	1,000 mg (M) 800 mg (F)	Carrots, broccoli, yams, dairy products, spinach	Antioxidant
B$_1$ Thiamine	1.5 mg (M)	Whole and enriched grain products, meat	Energy metabolism
B$_2$ Riboflavin	1.7 mg (M) 1.3 mg (F)	Dairy products, meat, leafy green vegetables	Energy metabolism
B$_3$ Niacin	20 mg (M)	Meat, enriched grain products, peanuts	Energy metabolism
B$_6$ Pyridoxine	2 mg	Whole grains, meat, fish, beans	Protein metabolism, red blood cells
B$_{12}$ Cobalamin	2 mcg	Meat, dairy products, fortified cereal	Cell metabolism, bone marrow, nervous system
Folic Acid	200–400 mcg	Leafy green veg., fruit, whole grains, veg's.	Red blood cells
Biotin	100–300 mcg	Dairy, whole grains	Energy metabolism
Pantothenic Acid	7–10 mg	Dairy products, whole grains, meat	Energy metabolism
C	60 mg	Citrus fruit, tomatoes, green veg., cantelope	Antioxidant, connective tissue, bones, vessels
D	5–10 mcg	Fish oil, milk, sunlight	Regulates calcium
E	7–13 mcg	Nuts, vegetable oil, green vegetables	Antioxidant, blood cell formation
K	65–80 mcg	Intestinal bacteria	Blood clotting
Calcium	800 mg (M) 1,200 mg (F)	Milk products, meat, grains, green veg's.	Teeth, bones, cell metabolism
Phosphorous	800 mg	Grains, meat, dairy	Energy metabolism
Iron	10 mg (M) 18 mg (F)	Liver, meat, whole and enriched grains	Red blood cells, energy metabolism
Zinc	15 mg	Beef, tuna, wheat, oatmeal, brown rice	Antioxidant, catalyst for metabolism
Selenium	100–200 mcg (not USRDA)	Tuna, chicken, dairy products	Antioxidant, related to vitamin E

* Beta-carotene is safer than vitamin A. USRDA is 20,000 International Units.

Then is a daily multivitamin all you need to take? Well, not quite. Current research indicates that beta carotene, vitamin E, and vitamin C are all helpful in deterring heart disease and cancer because of their role as antioxidants. They also help the immune system. Most multivitamins have these, but not enough. Take extra in the following amounts.

Beta-carotene	20,000 – 40,000 IUs per day
Vitamin E	400 – 800 milligrams per day
Vitamin C	500 milligrams per day

Quality vitamin supplements also contain the minerals calcium, potassium, phosphorous, iron, chlorine, and sulfur. Because the body is unable to make these minerals, which it incorporates into its bone, tissues, and fluids, they must be consumed. One mineral too easy to consume is sodium. Without it we cannot live. With too much of it, however, people with high blood pressure—at least 30 percent of our population—cannot live safely. If you have this condition, no doubt your doctor has told you to limit your salt intake. It's a prescription that's easier to dish out than it is to take. Most foods contain generous doses of salt, including sugar treats like colas and thick shakes. But don't get depressed over the prospect of a limited and tasteless diet. Exercise lowers blood pressure, which will allow you to use some salt.

One final note on vitamin supplements: do not link their acceptance to protein supplements. Frequently sold at health food stores, protein supplements are drastically overpriced and potentially dangerous. If you want protein, eat food; it costs less and tastes better.

Amid so much talk about vitamin and mineral supplements, it might seem that food plays only a supporting role in your diet. But food is always the star. You can't eat just anything, take vitamins, and live forever. A good diet is your life foundation, and it must follow you everywhere.

The Lowdown on "Sports Drinks"

Certainly an exercise program builds on a good diet. What you eat affects your energy level and even your heart rate. But there aren't many circumstances where you'll eat while exercising, unless of course, you're in a triathlon competition. Drinking is different.

You must drink during exercise, as well as before and after it. But that doesn't mean reaching for a specifically formulated sports drink. Gatorade, 10-K, Sportshot, Exceed—all vie for a piece of the market with promises of enhanced performance. What these drinks really enhance is their manufacturers' profits. They're expensive. For the money you spend you ought to get an enhanced performance; instead you get odd taste, a few tablespoons of sugar, and a smattering of electrolytes.

Electrolytes are the dissolved form of minerals. In sports drinks these minerals are sodium and potassium because these are excreted with sweat. Still, sweat is mostly water, and few minerals are lost even when fluid loss amounts to a quart. The only exercisers who need to replace electrolytes are endurance athletes whose daily workouts last at least three hours. But no sports drink contains enough potassium to replace what they've lost. They're better off eating bananas.

As for the sugar or carbohydrates in sports drinks, they too are unnecessary for most exercisers, and in some cases, such as when you want to lose weight, they undermine your effort. If you want to lose weight, you want to lose fat. Carbohydrates, when consumed immediately before and during a workout, become your body's energy of choice—instead of your fat stores. Even worse, after your body has used sports drink carbohydrates, it breaks into its own carbohydrate stores of muscle glycogen; the introduction of carbohydrates has encouraged the body to use more glycogen and less fat. It's as if the body is a car humming along in carbohydrate drive and it doesn't see the need to shift gears. So much for burning fat.

Sometimes, however, carbohydrates in drinks are handy. When you exercise intensely for over an hour, fluid loss through sweat can exceed a quart, and you must replace that as quickly as possible. Concentrations of carbohydrates below 8 percent speed up the intestines' absorption of water.

But first you must drink enough. Start drinking before you exercise: two to three cups one and one-half hours before and another cup one-half hour before. During your workout drink a half cup of water every 15 minutes, and afterward continue to drink as much as you can, especially if the weather is hot or the workout very intense.

That's a lot of drinking. Why not just depend on your thirst? The answer is that no parity exists between thirst and fluid loss;

thirst is satisfied long before lost fluids are replaced. Hence you don't drink enough because you're not thirsty enough and you get dehydrated.

Part of the problem with not drinking enough may be the drink itself. Bland tasting water doesn't exactly excite exercisers into drinking. What then can you drink if sports drinks taste lousy and water doesn't taste at all? To answer that, think back to your childhood. Do you remember a product called Kool-Aid®? Today it comes artificially sweetened and without calories in many delicious flavors. For especially drenching workouts, add some carbohydrates by taking a quart of artificially sweetened drink, replacing a cup of it with water and adding 4 tablespoons of sugar and $1/2$ teaspoon of Morton's Lite salt. In fewer than 5 minutes you make a tasty drink for a super workout. But don't bypass this simple recipe and reach for some fruit juice thinking that it contains sugar too. Its carbohydrate concentration is too high—it has too much sugar—and concentrations above 8 percent slow down water absorption by the intestines. Exactly the opposite of what you need.

And never—never drink alcohol before, during or after a workout. I've seen beer given out after 10-Ks and marathons. Apparently the race organizers didn't realize that alcohol, a diuretic, causes you to lose more fluid than it delivers. If you are dehydrated, as people often are after a workout, the alcohol will have a more potent effect on your brain: a couple of beers after work may not affect your driving. After a workout they will.

FIGHTING FOR MARKET SHARE

It's one thing to read about good nutrition; it's quite another to practice it. The interplay between nutrients and vitamins and the human body is complex, but I will simplify it with a business analogy. Think of food as a product produced and sold in the marketplace where there are three players: fats, proteins, and carbohydrates.

Today fat is the market leader with a 45 percent share, followed distantly by carbohydrates at 30 percent, and protein with the smallest share at 25 percent. (See Figure 11.3.) Your objective, as the company that produces carbohydrates, is to unseat fat as the leader and become number one, establishing the absolute dominance of

Figure 11.3	CALORIES		
Nutrient	Calories per Gram	% of Total Daily Calories	
		Current	Goal
Fat	9	45	25
Protein	4	25	15
Carbohydrates	4	30	60

Note: Water is excluded when calculating the percent of calories from each nutrient.

carbohydrates' market share. The market composition that will maximize the value of your company is carbohydrates at 60 percent, fat at 25 percent, and protein at 15 percent. What strategy will you use?

Before developing a plan, get some background from your Planning Department. The food market trades in calories instead of dollars for currency, so market share is measured in percent of calories. This gives fat the advantage because its "price" is 9 calories per gram, while protein's and carbohydrate's prices are only 4. All three producers use a daily accounting period to coincide with the consumer's biological need for their products. Each day they calculate their market share by multiplying the total volume of food—grams of fat, protein, and carbohydrates—by their price (9, 4, 4), and then dividing that product into their total sales.

At a time when value is the consumer's priority, it doesn't make sense that he would put up with fat's exorbitant price—and yet he does. One reason is that it tastes good. Many consumers have grown up with the taste and continue to crave it. Another reason is that they don't know they are buying it: people tend to categorize foods in terms of one nutrient. But most foods contain all three. A hamburger bun, for example, contains more than just carbohydrates; it contains protein and fat too. And look at pasta, the favorite carbohydrate of marathoners. Twenty percent of it is protein. The point is, if you want to get consumers more interested in your carbohydrate product, you must convince them to think of food as a combination of nutrients. Only then will they identify the expensive fat they are buying and cut back in favor of carbohydrates.

That's a logical strategy, but how do you implement it? Can you expect consumers to keep records of everything they eat, and then somehow dissect each food to uncover its fat content? No. To the consumer, time is also money, and this would be a waste of time. Therefore launch a major advertising campaign that urges the consumer to read labels. Government regulations require labels to expose the fat content of food. If consumers scan labels, they can comparison shop, noting that fat accounts for half the calories in product A and only one-fourth the calories in product B, and choose product B because it's less fat costly. Usually carbohydrates replace fat, so the less fat a product has, the more carbohydrates it must have.

Of course, you can expect the consumer to cut down on fat's market share, but you cannot expect the consumer to give it up altogether. This would be an unrealistic projection. Just expect consumers to eat fatty foods less often. Therein lies the secret to a healthier bottom line: a healthier consumer eats carbohydrates often and fats less often.

Increasing carbohydrate's market share from 30 percent to 60 percent cannot be done overnight. In the business world, a "quick fix" strategy like drastic price cutting can lead to a price war where everyone loses profits, but where the present market leader ultimately gets stronger. The same goes for nutritional fitness: a drastic strategy is doomed to failure. To succeed, you must change consumer preference gradually. You must also offer a superior product. Carbohydrates are already superior to fats—you just have to market them better. Emphasize carbohydrates; de-emphasize fats. Get the consumer to eat a superior product.

• CHAPTER 12 •

EVERYDAY EATING STRATEGIES

Bob and Judy work for the same large corporation, Bob as a regional sales manager and Judy as a public relations director. They are masters at juggling conflicts in their busy schedules, each sharing the responsibilities of running a home and raising their son and daughter. But when it comes to eating, their top priority is not nutrition. It's convenience. Breakfast is usually frantic: the kids eating their favorite cereal or a Pop Tart, Bob has coffee and a sausage biscuit in his car, and Judy eats a muffin or piece of fruit at her desk. Lunch means the office cafeteria for Judy and the school cafeteria for the children. Bob usually eats in restaurants while he sells to customers or networks with local office employees. Dinner is all over the map at one fast-food restaurant or another. There never seems to be enough time to cook at home.

In many households work schedules create a situation that pits time against eating, and eating usually loses. It leaves many a professional and executive with a daunting question: How can my family and I eat nutritiously without wasting too much time?

THREE MEALS A DAY

Eating nutritiously means eating carbohydrates, fat, and protein in the right proportions. Of course vitamins, minerals, fiber, and cholesterol play their roles as well. And all must be consistently eaten over the long run. In the realm of good nutrition, infrequent spates of conscientious eating do you little good. To eat properly in the long term, you must establish some basic eating habits on a daily basis.

It's better to eat three lighter meals a day than one or two bigger meals. Scientifically speaking, it may even be better to eat light snacks intermittently throughout the day, rather than three meals, but finding the right snacks, monitoring the right proportions of nutrients, and fighting the cultural current of three meals a day would be frustrating, stressful, and just not practical.

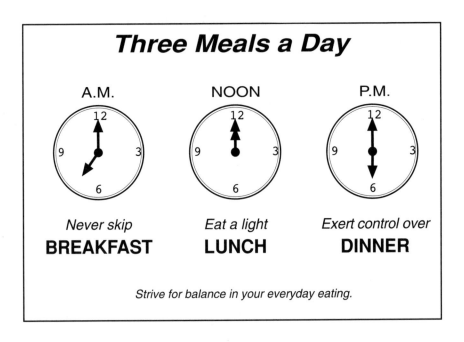

Three Meals a Day

A.M.   NOON   P.M.

Never skip **BREAKFAST**   *Eat a light* **LUNCH**   *Exert control over* **DINNER**

Strive for balance in your everyday eating.

Brighten Your Day with Breakfast

Let's say it's morning and you're in a rush to get to work. You can either eat a quick breakfast at home or pick up something on the way—those are the options most people will choose between. But the more important choice is the attitude you take toward this situation or any other time-short eating occasion. Will you just grab a quick bite—a donut, danish, or Pop Tart—so you don't feel starved or worry about your stomach growling during the 9:00 A.M. meeting? Or will you stop the frantic activity for a few moments and think of a way to eat a quick, nutritious breakfast, for example, a very lightly buttered bagel or a bowl of cereal with some skim milk?

It may surprise you that the habit of gulping an unhealthy breakfast—no fiber, no vitamins, too much fat and sugar—actually costs you time. This stance is supported by years of research that showed that unhealthy breakfasts impaired the performance of school children. The same applies to adults. Invest a few extra minutes on breakfast. Eat a cup of yogurt or a bowl of cereal before you leave, supplement that with a bagel and a cup of coffee on the way to work, and you'll be sharper all morning. The bottom line: you'll get more done.

A nutritious breakfast gives you a higher energy level and a better mental outlook, which improves your attitude toward work. It also prevents hunger later in the day, the time when most overeating occurs, and research even suggests that it helps people avoid eating fatty foods and snacking impulsively from the vending machine around the corner.

Light, Healthy Lunches Give You More Stamina

To many executives, lunch time is a signal to eat a large meal in a restaurant or cafeteria. But eating a big meal is not refreshing. In fact it slows you down. Normally your body's circadian rhythms slow you down at around 2:00 P.M. Why hasten that phase with a large meal? If you're a big lunch person, gradually introduce light lunches into your routine. How long this takes depends on your eating habits, but conservatively allow several months before completing the transition to light lunches every day.

To guarantee a light lunch that you enjoy, make it yourself. In some situations you might feel that brown bagging doesn't fit your style. Bluntly stated, it's too unprofessional. Let's dispel this misconception forever. Brown bagging shows the initiative to eat properly at all times—that you care about your health. Will this vigilant attitude go unnoticed in an era when health costs are skyrocketing toward the ionosphere? No. In fact companies are looking for just this kind of employee to promote as an example to other employees. Forget about that old impression that you're brown bagging because you're too cheap to buy your lunch. Health is in, extravagance is out.

The food industry has come a long way in supplying low-fat, low-calorie lunch options, and a small refrigerator in your office will give you the flexibility to use those options. Stock it with low-fat yogurts, skim milk and diet soda, cold salads and fat-free dressings, and sandwiches made with lean meats, fat-free cheeses, or water-packed tuna and fat-free mayonnaise.

Without a refrigerator you have fewer options, but don't give up. Store foods that require refrigeration in insulated bags chilled by a frozen gel pack. Commonly offered in mail order catalogs, these bags get food where it's going and can keep it chilled there all day. Or use the freeze-thaw trick. Freeze a container of low-fat yogurt and by noon it will be thawed and still cold. You can also freeze sandwiches. Cheeses, poultry, and sliced meats freeze well; mayonnaise and vegetable fillers don't.

Hot foods such as soups, stews, or casseroles stay well in thermoses. But make sure it's a good quality thermos that keeps the food hot, not just warm. When food is held warm, bacteria can multiply in hours.

Diet hot chocolate mix comes in safe, convenient single-serving packets. Just tap into the tea hot water supply at work and you have a drink that tastes as rich and chocolatey as the real thing—maybe better. Reach for this when you feel your sweet tooth beginning to stir. It's a hot drink that's satisfying enough to head off a candy bar snack.

Bringing your own lunches to work eliminates the wasted time of getting to and from a cafeteria or restaurant and waiting for service. You take the mystery out of whether your lunch is light and nutritious or hiding unwanted fat and calories, and you eliminate exposure to those weak moments of impulsively devouring a tasty appetizer, side order, or dessert.

Dinner Doesn't Have to Be Big and Fat

Traditionally, dinner has been the biggest meal of the day—big in terms of calories and time. Executives think in terms of using their

time efficiently and have turned to fast foods, cafeterias, steak hous-
es, and take-out food as the quickest way of eating dinner. This is
false economy. You save a little time on food preparation and waste
much more of it on traveling to the restaurant and waiting to be
served. As more and more busy people choose this way of eating, it
gets more and more crowded—on the roads and in the restaurants.
Eating out doesn't mean eating fast. It does mean losing control over
what's in the food you eat. In many restaurants it's virtually impossible to track the carbohydrates, fat, and protein in food someone else
prepares. All you can do is assume you're getting more fat than you
think as restaurants typically opt for taste over health.

Recently a professional working mother and acquaintance of
mine was trying to help her daughter with an interesting school
assignment: get the nutritional breakdown of menu items served at
Bob Evans family restaurant. Other classmates were assigned
McDonald's and Burger King. They were lucky. McDonald's, Burger
King, and other quick-serve giants have adopted a policy of full
nutrition disclosure. But Bob Evans' personnel didn't have any on
hand, and judging by how uncooperative they were with the stu-
dent, they didn't want to get it. If I were a Bob Evans' manager, I
wouldn't tell the public how much fat is in the sausage gravy either.
(See Figure 12.1 for the fat content of some popular foods.)

TAKE FULL CONTROL OF YOUR NUTRITIONAL FITNESS

For many, eating at home carries a stigma. Some people think it's
boring, some think it wastes time, and some just hate cooking. You
work hard all day. Why should you cook when you get home?

Obviously, you must make some effort to eat at home, but the
advantages far outstrip the energy expended. Take breakfast, for
example. Research shows that homemade breakfasts average 6 percent less fat than typical breakfasts eaten out. Extend that point
beyond breakfasts to include lunch, dinner, and snacks too. Here,
control is a critical factor. When you prepare a dish yourself, you
have complete control over what goes in it, and if not—some of the
ingredients are already semiprocessed—you at least know exactly
what's in them because of government-sponsored labeling. How
many restaurant meals do you have that much control over?

Figure 12.1   **FAT CONTENT OF SOME POPULAR FOODS**

	Calories	Fat (g)	% Calories from Fat
Breakfast			
OVER 25%			
Sausage/egg biscuit	520	34	59
Donut	170	11	58
Buttermilk biscuit	235	12	46
Oat bran muffin	430	20	42
French toast	153	7	41
UNDER 25%			
Oatmeal (3/4 cup)	102	2	18
Pancakes (Aunt Jemima Lite)	140	2	13
English muffin	135	1	7
Plain bagel	163	1	6
Corn flakes (w/ skim milk)	140	0	0
Lunch			
OVER 25%			
Taco Light	411	29	64
Big Mac	560	33	53
Nachos	356	19	48
Hot dog	260	14	48
Plain pizza (Pizza Hut)	520	20	35
UNDER 25%			
Tuna sandwich (low-fat mayo)	300	7	21
Bologna (low-fat) sandwich	240	4	15
Turkey sandwich	213	3	13
Yogurt (vanilla)	210	3	13
Cheese (no-fat) sandwich	240	2	8
Dinner			
OVER 25%			
Pork chops (roasted)	515	28	49
Meatloaf	525	26	45
New York strip steak	550	27	44
Fried chicken	590	27	41
Roast beef	460	16	31
UNDER 25%			
Red snapper (baked)	385	10	23
Shrimp (steamed)	350	8	21
Lobster (boiled)	350	8	21
Spaghetti	500	9	16

Dinners (except spaghetti) include 4 ounces of meat, baked potato, green beans, and two pats of butter.

The Convenience of Frozen Dinners

As for the time factor, with some planning eating in, which includes cooking, takes less time than eating out. First decide what meals you are going to make. Next have all the ingredients on hand. Repeated trips to the supermarket are enough to convince anyone to eat out, but they can be avoided by making a list when you plan the meals. After eating, don't throw away leftovers and don't relegate them to a dark corner of the refrigerator where they'll just grow mold. Plan to use them in the future by labeling and freezing them.

Speaking of freezing food, the ultimate leftovers are what you cook in bulk to be frozen for future dinners. Most soups, stews, and casseroles freeze well. So do sliced meats like turkey breast or lean ham.

Chapter 8, "Take-Home Fitness," describes a wide variety of exercise equipment that can make your cardio and muscular fitness goals easier and more convenient to achieve. Other than the standard kitchen equipment, the single most convenient piece of equipment I can think of to help achieve your nutritional fitness goals is a full-size upright freezer. An upright freezer is better than a chest freezer because it's easier to organize and provides ready access to most items. If you don't think you need another freezer, in addition to the small one with your refrigerator, think about the times you moved into a larger house or apartment. In no time at all, the additional closet and storage space in the new home became occupied. The same is true of a second freezer. It will become so full of so many different meals (see Figure 12.2) that choosing dinner will be like deciding which restaurant to go to, but with more convenience and control. Remember, this is your cooking, not someone else's.

I realize that this advice may leave some cooking-shy professionals disheartened. "Isn't there another way to eat 'at home' without cooking up a storm?" they ask. To answer that question I send them down the frozen food aisles. Gone are the days when these aisles served as shelf space for bland-tasting TV dinners and monotonous frozen vegetables. Today they are crammed with a variety of tastier frozen dinners—the marketplace's response to the consumer's hectic schedule.

But don't trust everything on those icy shelves. Frozen dinners offer the ultimate in convenience, some also offer the ultimate in fat, calories and salt. Look at the fat content of frozen dinners. About

Figure 12.2	FREEZE FOR CONVENIENCE
Premade Meals	**Other Foods That Freeze Well**
Spaghetti sauce	Sandwich bread, buns
Vegetable soup	Assorted vegetables (cooked)
Chile	Gravies (low-fat)
Beef, chicken, pork stew	Stuffings
Turkey slices	Waffles
Turkey tetrazzini	Ham slices (center cut)
Hot dogs (low-fat)	Baked goods (no-fat)
Chicken cacciatore	English muffins
Hamburger patties (lean)	Berries

half the calories in most deep fried chicken and fish entrees are from fat. That's too much.

Before you choose any dinner, read the label for its fat content, calorie count, nutrients and weight. Though these dinners are prepared by someone else, at least you'll know the ingredients they used. Chicken and fish entrees are usually low fat if they are not fried or swimming in a cream sauce. Pasta entrees sans cream and butter sauces are also good choices. But don't expect them to fill you. Most frozen dinners have the airline meal syndrome—they don't contain enough food to satisfy a normal appetite—and most aren't nutritionally balanced.

To solve these common problems add to the meals your own easy-to-make side dishes. Easiest to make and most nutritious are frozen vegetables. The freezer section is well stocked with tasty vegetable combinations, far more appealing than the bags of one kind only and just as easy to make. But not all frozen vegetables are suitable as meal stretchers. Any vegetables residing in a bag with butter or cream sauce leave in the freezer case. Along with them leave vegetables that come with spice packets and directions to add butter or margarine. Frozen vegetables mean frozen vegetables only. To retain most of their nutrients cook them in the microwave or a covered pot with a small amount of water, none of which is left when they're finished cooking. I add some butter substitute and a touch of onion powder and chicken broth to give vegetables a richer flavor.

Microwaving

Like most kitchens, yours is probably equipped with a microwave oven. This is truly a gift to a time-scarce society. Not since I watched the Jetsons have I seen a device that could cook as fast. But how many people really cook in it? What's more likely is that you use it for peripheral cooking duties: defrosting and reheating. Fish and chicken cooked in the microwave without added fat come out tender and delicious, and so do vegetables. In fact I heard about a woman who cooked her entire Thanksgiving dinner—turkey, stuffing, yams, peas, and acorn squash—in it. I'm not recommending that you perform such a feat with your microwave. Just that you use it as more than a popcorn popper.

Broiling

Another fat fighter is your broiler. Broiling is a dry heat method of cooking that requires the most tender—which also means the fattiest—cuts of beef or pork, and therefore would seem to be a method to avoid. But like the microwave, the broiler cooks without adding fat, and it allows indigenous fat to drip away. So how do you broil tougher, less fatty cuts of meat? You marinate them, preferably overnight in the refrigerator or for one hour at room temperature. By marinate, I mean placing the meat in an acidic liquid, like teriyaki sauce or a low-fat salad dressing, not in a fatty marinade that will coat and permeate the meat with oil. Most marinade recipes contain more oil than necessary.

Simmering

Even your stove and oven have much potential as low-fat cookers. In both you can moist cook any meat by submerging one-third of it in liquid, tightly covering the pot or pan, and simmering it just below a boil. Moist cooking has two advantages. It tenderizes tougher cuts of meat, which contain less fat, and it requires no fat to be added. How long you moist cook meat, which depends on its size and cut, is information any all-purpose cookbook will give you. But remember, the liquid you cook it in must be low fat or you might as well fry it.

Moist cooking also yields delicious low-fat gravies. But when meat trimmed of fat cooks in water, it flavors the water only delicately, probably not enough to make a robust gravy. Therefore reinforce any gravies with the relevant broth, for example, a chicken broth for a chicken or turkey gravy. Add butter substitute for a richer flavor, some flour or potato flakes to thicken it, and you have a first-rate gravy.

Frying

From these cooking tips it may seem as if I never, God forbid, use a frying pan. At times, however, I do and so will you. This is a fact of cooking, but it needn't be an unhealthy one if your skillet has a nonstick surface and you prime it with a thin layer of vegetable spray before cooking.

Frying pans aren't the only cooking utensils that come with a nonstick coating. Griddles, waffle irons, and sandwich cookers also have nonstick cooking surfaces. Take advantage of them by using little or no fat—they don't need it. Don, an architect and careful eater, recently told me about the pancakes he had at an old-fashioned diner during a business trip. They were cooked on what looked like an ancient griddle, and as he watched dollops of shortening melt on that griddle, he realized what kind of breakfast he was about to eat: a greasy one. Unlike his homemade pancakes, which are cooked on a nonstick griddle without fat, these pancakes were fried—so fried that their edges were crispy. Don will not be ordering pancakes at diners anymore.

Don't look at cooking as drudgery. What we're all striving for—what we want to believe that we have—is control over our lives. Food is certainly a part of our lives that we can control. Think of cooking as a creative activity that gives us the ultimate control.

STRATEGIES FOR EATING OUT

Eating out has become more than a national pastime; it's a way of life. Is this a problem? Yes—it's a threat to our health. "When we eat out, we eat too much," wrote an experienced editor of a national health magazine. Since 1965 the money spent on food prepared outside the home has risen over 625 percent. That statistic matches recent surveys that say the average family now eats out over 50 percent of the time, and that doesn't include breakfasts, lunches, and dinners eaten during the course of business. For these business meals, we also see an increase: restaurant deliveries to offices are up 30 percent over the last decade—not to mention the lunches and dinners with clients or the Friday lunches out to herald the coming weekend.

Full-Service Restaurants

The most seductive eating out scenario unfolds when you travel on business. There you are at some hotel, perhaps a bit bored, perusing the room service menu or asking the desk clerk for the names of good restaurants in the city. Money is no object or not much of an object; you're armed with an expense account. These are the circumstances that lead to the most lavish eating.

Lavish or not, it is better to leave the hotel, or at least your room, to have dinner. Room service is the ultimate trap. In general it has a more limited menu than the hotel restaurant, though any entrees common to both menus are identical: a steak ordered from room service is cooked in the same kitchen as a steak ordered in the restaurant. But ordering from room service isn't the same. What it doesn't offer that the hotel restaurant does—besides three times the entrees—is the advantage of person-to-person communication. To eat a balanced, low-fat meal out, you must know how to order. You must also have the cooperation of the waiter. With room service you get an anonymous voice over the phone, someone who doesn't have to face you when the meal is delivered or when the tip is decided. All the ordering savvy in the world won't overcome that disadvantage.

ASK QUESTIONS. When dining at a full-service restaurant always ask questions. This is no time to be bashful. Restaurants are selling a product and a service. The product is cooked food. The service is cooking that food. Therefore, employees of restaurants should be able to answer your questions. If possible, call ahead with a polite and inquisitive attitude. In today's atmosphere of healthful disclosure, most restaurant personnel should respond positively to your needs, explaining how the menu items are prepared and listening carefully to how you want it changed. Nearly 70 percent of the restaurant managers surveyed by MasterCard said it was all right to ask for a menu switch. The National Restaurant Association agrees. It estimates that 8 out of 10 restaurants would, upon request, bake or broil food instead of frying it and skin chicken before cooking it. Take advantage of this trend.

Add to the inquisitive approach an understanding of menu lingo. Descriptions like steamed, poached, broiled, and cooked in its own juices suggest that the cooking method is a low-fat one. Pan fried, sautéed, rich, and crisp, on the other hand, tell you it's high in fat.

Some restaurant menus are sporting little red hearts. Posted beside supposedly low-fat entrees, these little hearts carry an air of authority even though they don't conform to any government guidelines that define exactly what they mean. Presumably that is left to the chef. One Sunday I watched a prominent Louisiana chef cook a duck by simmering it in fat rendered from its own skin. Would you trust this man's definition of low fat? Fortunately, in more and more restaurants, chefs are rising to the occasion. No longer must they rely on butter or fat as a shortcut to good taste. Demand has forced them to create different flavorings using herbs, and stocks of beef, chicken, and vegetables. Nowadays many chefs consider a low-fat request a challenge to their skill and creativity.

Are you ready to order?

APPETIZERS/SALADS. Let's assume you've called ahead to make sure restaurant management has a cooperative attitude toward special requests, and now you're seated at a table in the restaurant reading the menu. What should you order for an appetizer? Wise choices include fruit cups and raw vegetables, steamed seafood and shrimp cocktail in cocktail sauce, tomato-based soups and clear broths, including french onion soup without cheese. Avoid breaded or battered appetizers; they're fried and therefore high in fat. Also avoid creamed soups, patés, and fish immersed in cream sauce.

Salads that are served to you shouldn't present a problem. Nine in ten restaurant owners surveyed said they would gladly serve any salad dressing or sauce on the side. If they serve a low-calorie dressing, choose that, but dribble it on your salad cautiously because these "house-made" dressings may not be as low in fat as what you can buy at the supermarket. In fact supermarkets sell certain brands of dressings in single serving packets. These would be your best choices.

Salad bars are increasingly popular and almost every salad bar is loaded with enough high-fat items to turn an innocent salad into a wicked dish. Still, they do offer low-fat foods. Just avoid the bacon bits and the chopped eggs, the cheeses and the sunflower seeds, the chow mein noodles, and all the mayonnaise-laced salads.

Along with salads usually come rolls or bread. Breads, especially whole grains, are excellent low-fat foods, but in restaurants butter or margarine is always their sidekick. Use it very sparingly and never accept prebuttered bread. Restaurant personnel think you want a ton of butter, and maybe in the past you did. But that was then; this is now. Inform them otherwise.

ENTREES. Be discriminating when you select the meat in your entree. Fish, skinless chicken, and turkey contain the least fat. Prime beef contains the most, much of it saturated. But not all beef dishes may be prime. Before you order beef, ask what grades they serve; do they have any dishes made with choice or select grades? Remember prime beef is a prime example of a nutritional disaster.

Also remember that you are in a full-service restaurant, where you have the most say. Ask how the entree is cooked. If it's not grilled, broiled, poached, or steamed, see if it can be cooked with any of those methods. Request that grilling or broiling be done "dry" so your meat doesn't get basted in fat. If the entree has a special sauce added during cooking, ask for the sauce to be served on the side. Always be as specific as possible. Don't just ask the waiter for a "low-fat version" of your entree; tell him how you want it made low fat, leaving only the finer points of cooking to the chef.

One detail the waiter won't leave to the chef is how well done you want your meat cooked, as it is standard procedure to ask the patron that question in most full-service restaurants. Never order meat rare. As meat cooks it loses fat. When you shorten the cooking time, you literally leave behind the fat that would have eventually cooked out. Another thing you might want to leave behind is any excess portion. Typically restaurants give much more protein than you need. Try to order a petite serving, or a children's serving, or an appetizer portion of meat if you can.

Where restaurants overload you in protein, they short you in vegetables. Vegetables are usually the handmaidens of protein, scattered sparsely around it on the plate or sitting meekly off to the side in a separate dish. But they deserve more respect and attention. When steamed or microwaved, vegetables are nutrient dense and very low in fat and calories. Butter them, or even worse, cream them, and you drown the nutrients in fat and calories. In the world of restaurants, vegetables are no safe harbor. Follow your normal ordering technique of asking how they are prepared and what size portion you will be getting. If fat is added, request the vegetables be served without it. If the serving size is small, order a double portion. Don't leave yourself hungry for dessert.

DESSERTS. Good restaurants are expert in making their desserts look delicious. Daintily decorated with everything from fruit to nuts, these filthy rich treats wait patiently for you to finish your entree and order them. Will you order your usual cheesecake or that outrageous chocolate torte you've been staring at all evening? One of the most memorable features of a business meal I ate at the Four Seasons in New York was its dessert tray. All evening I stared at it—some of the desserts I couldn't even identify—and at the end of the meal I ordered what must have been the richest, densest piece of chocolate cake on earth.

Don't torture yourself or weaken your willpower. If a dessert cart is within view, ask the waiter to move it away, explaining that you'd like to avoid the temptation. If it's not visible, make sure the waiter knows not to bring it around at the end of the meal. And never let yourself be seated next to a dessert display that doesn't move. From your table you'd like a pleasant view—a postcard sunset or nighttime city skyline.

Cafeterias

Cafeterias, smorgasbords, and restaurant buffets are not as common as full-service restaurants and it's a good thing; all their dishes are prepared in advance, giving you absolutely no control over the cooking method or ingredients. What you do have control over is what entree you choose and perhaps the amount of salad dressing and gravy you get. Or do you? Avoiding fat is hard enough without this sumptuous setup shaking your willpower—only the most stalwart eater won't succumb. If you have any say in where you eat, choose another—any other—kind of restaurant.

Airlines

The airline industry is fiercely competitive. Its business is transporting people—mostly business travelers—and food service is just another cost center. What it serves doesn't have to be healthy for the masses, who are after all, a captive audience; it has to be edible—not a very high standard for a major restaurant chain of the business world.

As a business traveler you may not be very concerned about what airlines serve, preferring instead to dine at restaurants on land, but tight schedules may make eating in the air necessary at times. In that case, beware. Much of what airlines serve is high in fat and low in bulk—lots of calories and little food. But most airlines also offer special meals that are low in salt, fat, or cholesterol if you request them at least 48 hours before the flight departs. Get in the habit of doing this when you book your flight and confirm that the airline has it recorded when you check in.

A special meal might solve your fat and calorie problem, but it won't satisfy your hunger. Airline meals are notoriously skimpy. Prepare yourself for that by bringing along your own bulk, some fruit, or pretzels, or even a sandwich, so when the flight attendant offers you those salty peanuts, you won't even want them.

Finally, never order a cocktail in the air. As I have always insisted, alcohol has no place in a healthy diet, and even less of a place at 30,000 feet. The friendly skies can get awfully turbulent. Alcohol especially can give you a throat tightening, unsettled feeling, as a woman sitting near me found out on a flight to Cincinnati. Her Bloody Mary promptly resurfaced after we hit some minor turbulence. Keep your exact change.

Fast Foods

Fast-food restaurants outnumber all other kinds of restaurants and their revenues easily exceed $50 billion a year. That's millions of hamburgers, pizzas, and fried chickens. These are the foods that appeal to the kids, and kids often influence what their parents eat, which is why even executives end up ordering in them.

But asking the employees of some of these restaurants for nutritional information will get you nowhere. It's up to you to look for low-fat fare. During a breakfast stop choose plain bagels or English muffins (easy on the butter), plain pancakes with syrup only, cereals with low-fat (or preferably skim) milk, or any low-fat muffin. For lunch or dinner, eat salads with "lite" dressings, turkey or roast beef sandwiches, regular hamburgers, plain baked or mashed potatoes, or corn on the cob. If you crave pizza, order one with the thickest crust and the least cheese. Or, better still, order a veggie pizza without cheese. Drink diet soda, black coffee, or skim milk. Forget dessert—unless it's McDonald's superb frozen yogurt.

Bypassing dessert is one thing, pretending that your favorite high-fat meal isn't waiting to be ordered is another. If you must have an old favorite, disarm it at least partially by asking them to hold the cheese, mayonnaise, or tartar sauce. If that changes the meal too much for your taste buds, try a more liberal approach. Order the sandwich and remove most of the dressing yourself, leaving just enough for a hint of flavor. Use the same trick for sandwiches topped with bacon or for chicken or fish coated with a fried batter or breading. Remove the bacon or the coating. Some of its flavor will remain.

Instead of knowing what to order or how to make it accept-able, a different strategy is knowing what to avoid. In the fast-food world there's plenty. No matter what restaurant you eat in, avoid menu items with biscuits, croissants, sausage, bacon, cheese (except pizza), and pepperoni. Also off limits are cookies, danish, donuts, pies, and gourmet ice creams. That sounds like a good portion of any fast-food menu and it is. Unfortunately it's not all inclusive. Identify the rest of these food demons by their names. Consider any menu item described with words like Big and Jumbo, Double and Deluxe, Ultimate and Supreme, Extra, Fried, Cheese or Platter untouchable. (See Figure 12.3 for a summary of eating strategies.)

Figure 12.3	**STRATEGIES FOR EATING OUT**
Full-Service Restaurants	Ask questions about low-fat options and cooking methods. Beware of salad bar toppings. Order small meat portions. Avoid desserts.
Cafeterias	Find another option. You have no control over the ingredients or cooking method. The clever food displays destroy your willpower.
Airlines	Order special meals in advance. Supplement them with your own fruit, pretzels, or even a home-made sandwich.
Fast Foods	Shop for low-fat alternatives. Avoid entrees named Jumbo, Deluxe, Supreme, Extra, Fried, Cheese, and Platter.

Where you choose to eat will determine the degree of control you have over your nutrition fitness. Eating food that you prepare gives you complete control over its ingredients. Eating food prepared by someone else gives you less control, but it doesn't leave you helpless. Ultimately the choices and decisions are in your hands. Make them wisely or lose control not only of what you eat, but also of what you weigh.

• CHAPTER 13 •

CONTROLLING YOUR WEIGHT

Tracy is considered to be on the "fast track" in the well-known consulting firm where she works. And work she does. Proud of her persistence and workaholic mind-set, Tracy is convinced that these are two important ingredients of success. She is also aware that a professional appearance is another ingredient and that extra weight hurts her chances of making partner. For Tracy, controlling her weight may be her greatest professional challenge. Ever since her teenage years she has struggled with her weight and is a veteran of many quick weight-loss schemes. Tracy didn't mind the suffering and arduous labor of complying with those diets—not if it accomplished something as worthwhile as weight loss. So she went on diets that in no way resembled how she ate. She made those odd-tasting recipes. She ate the grapefruits, the carrots, the celery. But like many dieters who succeed in losing some weight, the success is always fleeting. She keeps gaining the weight back again.

Tracy's not alone. A recent poll found that 61 percent of adults were overweight. It's a sad statistic, considering that their chances of losing that extra weight and keeping it off are almost nil. Fewer than 57 percent of dieters ever reach their ideal weight, and 90 percent of those that do gain the weight back. This translates into a suc-

223

cess rate of less than five percent. It's a cure rate lower than cancer's.

These dismal statistics don't even tell the whole sad story. As a refugee of diets, not only have you gained back any weight you lost; you've gained more and, at the same time, made it easier for yourself to gain body fat. All this at the risk of your health.

TODAY'S DIETS AREN'T WORKING

Why such profound failure in a time when best-selling diets abound? Because a diet doesn't have to work to sell; it just has to offer hope— which is what millions of people like Tracy keep reaching for. But this hope is false. Today's diets, including such well-known ones as the Cambridge, the Scarsdale, the Pritikin, the Nutrisystem, the T Factor, the Slimfast, the Hilton Head, and the Jenny Craig, don't work because they have two fundamental flaws: the food you eat is not "yours," and the reward for success is inappropriate.

Almost every diet disregards a person's food preferences. Oh, they claim to offer a wide variety of foods from which to choose, but somehow it never feels that way when you're eating them. In fact it feels as if you are living in a car with all the foods allotted to you stashed in the glove compartment. Your eating habits and preferences aren't even shared by members of your family, let alone people from all over the country. To tell you to lose weight by forcing yourself to eat specific foods is to tell a top executive to take an extended vacation. It won't work. Radically changing your normal eating habits and tolerating it for a limited time is futile and foolish. Willpower and suffering don't guarantee permanent weight loss.

The second flaw is in the reward. With most diets, your reward for suffering through their restrictive regimens is weight loss. Suppose you do make it to your target weight. What is going to keep you there? Without the goal of weight loss to reach for, you'll find yourself reaching for danish, donuts, and candy bars. From there your only direction is up—that is in weight.

With flaws like these it's no wonder today's diets aren't working. OptimEating, however, does work. It's new and it's different. OptimEating is not a diet, but a three-step plan to a lifelong way of eating that emphasizes getting the most pleasure out of calories you consume.

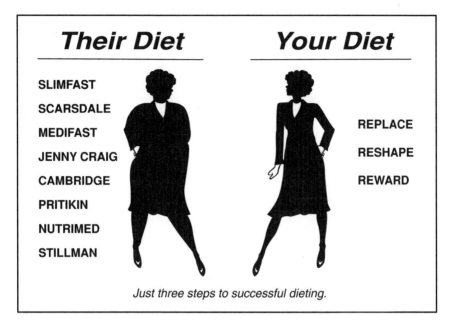

Their Diet	Your Diet
SLIMFAST	
SCARSDALE	
MEDIFAST	REPLACE
JENNY CRAIG	RESHAPE
CAMBRIDGE	REWARD
PRITIKIN	
NUTRIMED	
STILLMAN	

Just three steps to successful dieting.

There is no suffering with strange foods, overwhelming portions, or fasting. You'll fashion new eating habits based on *your* food preferences. The first step is to REPLACE foods you currently eat with more nutritious variations. Specifically, you'll focus on replacing unhealthy fat with carbohydrates as your primary source of calories.

The second step is to RESHAPE bad eating habits into good ones. You'll learn tactics to break the eating momentum that leads to overindulging, to control the stimuli that weaken your willpower, and to eat well-balanced meals and healthy snacks routinely. To be safe and effective, this reshaping step applies proven behavioral conditioning techniques.

The third step, REWARD, ensures the permanency of OptimEating. There will be no more demoralizing weight fluctuations. You won't gain the weight back; you'll control it and reach a level of nutritional fitness you never dreamed possible by giving yourself an appropriate reward at the right time. You'll also enjoy eating more than ever before because your reward will be the very food you love most.

REPLACE FATS WITH CARBOHYDRATES

Step 1 eases you into your new way of eating without drastic calorie cuts or severe food restrictions. What you eat does not change, except for its composition. Here carbohydrates will take the place of fat. This accomplishes two things: it cuts calories and maintains your metabolic rate. The body expends more energy breaking down carbohydrates than it does breaking down fats, a processing inefficiency you want to take advantage of. Your mission is to decide what foods to replace.

Start by thinking about your diet. What fatty foods do you eat? Thanks to the government's new regulations on labeling, it shouldn't be hard to tell; just read labels. As you identify the foods, write them down. Then look over the list and pick out a few foods you can replace easily.

Don't immediately replace every food on the list; that would turn your diet upside down. To ensure success, you must avoid such a massive upheaval. Be patient. This may be the hardest part of the replacement phase. Once you make the decision to lose weight, it suddenly becomes an urgent goal, and the thought of doing it slowly annoys you. "Why replace a few foods at a time, when I can do the job in one fell swoop?" you might ask. The answer is if you do the job that way you won't finish it. Your body and your mind won't cooperate. By taking the gradual route, you'll make changes that last.

Nowadays some of the easiest foods to replace are dairy products. Milk, cheese, butter, yogurt, ice cream—all have excellent low-fat or fatless versions. But remember to ease into each replacement. Don't instantly replace a full-fat food with a fatless food. Take milk, for example. If you switch from whole milk to skim milk, you will probably think you are drinking cloudy water. Do it in stages: first switch to 2 percent milk, and then only after you are accustomed to 2 percent milk, switch to 1 percent milk. Eventually you will be drinking skim milk and enjoying it.

Another example is salad dressing. Say you use Thousand Island dressing, a product that comes in low-fat and fatless varieties. First get used to the low-fat variety. Then only after you're happy with the low-fat dressing—that shouldn't take long because its taste and texture are amazingly close to that of its fatty forebearer—switch to the fatless version.

When you have successfully replaced the first few foods, go back to your list and pick a few more. Keep repeating this cycle until you have replaced as many foods on the list as you can. For some items there won't be a like-kind replacement available. Sausage, for example, does come in "light" varieties, but these are still so fatty that they don't qualify as replacements.

In a case like this consider replacing breakfast sausage with another meat like Canadian bacon, which is different, but serves the same purpose: a meat for breakfast. And speaking of breakfast, perhaps you are one of the many people who buy it from fast-food restaurants. Here we go again with sausage, or maybe it's bacon and eggs. Whatever it is, it's a diet disaster, full of fat, much of it saturated. Some fast-food outlets do have low-fat alternatives. McDonald's, for example, has low-fat as well as fatless muffins. But many other restaurants do not. If the restaurant you go to doesn't, why not replace that fatty breakfast with cereal and skim milk. It provides plenty of protein, carbohydrates, and much more fiber than a greasy sandwich. Of course you can't eat cereal while you're driving, so wait until you get to the office and impress your coworkers with a decidedly healthy breakfast that is guaranteed to start your day better.

Replacing some of the foods on your list will depend on your own cooking skills. To look at the diet books sold today, you'd think that the world was made up of overweight gourmets just looking for unusual recipes to prepare. "I've never heard of a diet book without recipes," an editor once told me. "Dieters need recipes." This, of course, is not true. Dieters do not need new recipes; nor do they want them. Given the time constraints of executives, who perhaps juggle the responsibilities of a two-career family, of single parenthood, and of many other modern developments, cooking is an activity they don't have much time to do. Still, at some point, you must cook—but don't suffer through someone else's recipes. Simply "replace" the recipes you already use by defatting them through changes in ingredients and cooking methods.

A replacement food must taste good to you. Don't make substitutions that are terrible tasting or inconvenient. If a replacement doesn't work out, be patient and take heart: food manufacturers are on the job. I've tasted a fatless mayonnaise that was too bland only to discover six months later that the product was vastly improved. Be willing to try products again, to adjust a recipe more than once. One way or another, you've got to replace some foods in your diet. Use your curiosity and creativity to discover new products; you have plenty to work with. In 1981 supermarkets offered about 40 reduced-fat products. That figure soared to 1,260 by 1992. And more help is on the way.

Most important, keep an open mind and a positive attitude. Don't say: "I can't do it." "I'll never like it." "I won't put up with a different taste." These are defeatist attitudes. If you have a negative attitude about replacing any of your favorite foods—and denying it would be a fatal blow to your replacement endeavors—trick yourself with blind taste tests. For years my brother refused to try low-calorie pancake syrup. "That isn't real maple syrup," he'd say. So one morning we staged a blind taste test pitting 100 percent maple syrup against Log Cabin light. He chose the Log Cabin light.

The basic principle behind replacement is to find alternatives with fewer calories. (See Figure 13.1.) That carbohydrates are healthier for you than fat is important no matter what you weigh. If you're trying to lose weight, however, the bottom line is calories and the easiest way to avoid them is to replace fat with carbohydrates, which have five fewer calories per gram.

Some people take this message too literally. A year ago I was standing in line to pay in a drugstore, when I overheard a woman tell the cashier that her doctor wanted her to lose weight. "He told me to cut down on fat," she said, while placing a bag of fatless jelly beans on the counter. "So I've been eating these and I've already gained three pounds." In the business of weight loss it pays to invest in carbohydrates, but don't overextend yourself. The body turns excess calories—whether fat, protein, or carbohydrates—into fat, and there is no magic way to get around it.

RESHAPE Bad Eating Habits into Good Ones

A behaviorist describes changing eating habits as a complex task. To teach an animal a complex task, you must introduce pieces of that task over time, a technique called "shaping," and it is the only way

Figure 13.1	REPLACEMENT IDEAS
Milk	Use skim milk or 1% milk instead of whole milk or 2% milk.
Eggs	Replace whole eggs with Egg Beaters or egg whites. Two egg whites replace one whole egg.
Bread	Regular bread doesn't have much fat, but diet breads have half the calories and taste just as good.
Spreads	Use soft tub, light margarines instead of stick margarines or any kind of butter.
Bacon or Sausage	Canadian bacon or lean ham.
Lunch Meats	Choose any 97% fat-free replacements.
Pork Chop	Pork tenderloin and cut off all visible fat.
Beef	Turkey breast or fish marinated in teriyaki sauce.
Ground Beef	Sauté, drain, and rinse with hot water before using.
USDA Prime	USDA Choice or Select.
Poultry	Any light meat instead of dark meat.
Cheese	Replace full-fat cheeses with low- or no-fat varieties, including American, cottage, and cream cheeses.
Fats and Oils	In cooking recipes reduce oil by two-thirds. Use stronger-tasting olive oil to stretch flavor. Replace butter with butter flavor substitute. In baking recipes reduce fat by one-half and replace that fat with half as much corn syrup.

an animal can learn. The same applies to humans. But your vastly superior intellect is challenged by much more complex tasks, such as prying yourself loose from habits that have been psychologically and physiologically entrenched since childhood.

That's why drastic calorie cuts, as in many reputable diets, don't work. Your body interprets this change as a sudden food shortage, and it reacts by conserving energy with a slowdown of its metabolic rate. Of course, you don't realize this. What you do realize is that you have stopped losing weight. You also realize that you feel cold and irritable, and are unable to concentrate well—all signs of physiological withdrawal. As far as your body is concerned, the crash diet is the bad habit that must be replaced with heavier eating, and it screams to the brain to get it more food. The brain does this easily because it has the help of your old eating habits, which haven't changed—that reputable, best-selling diet never addressed them.

Both the mind and body fend off the unreasonable change demanded by a drastic diet with ferocious force, and instead of becoming nutritionally fit, you become a battle ground. Avoid this battle by changing gradually—that is, replace bad habits with good habits, one at a time. Taking one day at a time has been a pivotal strategy of Alcoholics Anonymous for years, but it is also a powerful strategy for loosening the vicelike grip of eating habits that have defeated you so many times in the past. It is very difficult to suddenly break a habit, thinking you can simply banish it from your life without some backlash. Instead, patiently reshape your habits. This gradual introduction suits the psychological as well as the physiological aspects of behavioral conditioning.

To reshape your eating habits, first ask yourself honestly, "What do I eat and when do I eat it?" and then list your answers. Executives, being a captive audience of the corporate atmosphere—especially other executives—tend to fall into the same bad eating habits, snacking on cookies and danish during meetings, overeating at lunch, indulging in cocktails and lavish business dinners, and snacking while working late or after they get home. Use the following strategies to reshape these harmful habits forever.

EAT BALANCED MEALS. For most people, the later in the day it is, the harder it is to change your eating habits. So start with the easiest, breakfast. Eating oat bran or any number of healthy breakfast cereals with skim milk is an excellent strategy to replace eggs, bacon, sausage, biscuits, or other fatty foods. Never skip breakfast. It has great potential to improve your nutritional fitness.

Morning snacks, on the other hand, can be eliminated, but not all at once. For example, if you indulge in a midmorning muffin, eat only half, stretching it with a cup of tea or coffee. Don't mindlessly gobble it down during a phone conversation, and don't leave the other half in sight to tempt you.

After reshaping your morning habits, you are ready to downsize lunch. A big lunch takes your mind off work. Other than that, it works heartily against you, producing lethargy, impairing concentration, and decreasing motivation—in short, lowering your productivity. Minimize it; avoid alcohol, large entrees, and desserts. A light lunch is a power lunch.

As for afternoon snacks or any snacks for that matter, overcome them by procrastinating. If you have a daily snack that puts pounds on you and interferes with your work, drop it. But not in one day. First, delay it 15 minutes each day for several days. Next, lengthen the delay to 30 minutes, then 45 minutes. Eventually the snack will end up so close to a meal that it will become obsolete.

The most challenging reductions are those made later in the day. Food's pull increases as the day winds down. Whether it's because you're hungry or tired or anxious is unimportant; overeating at night is the downfall of many an executive, and it requires aggressive and confrontational tactics to stop it.

CONTROL FOOD STIMULI. Research studies confirm that exposure to food alone can significantly weaken willpower. Though there is not much you can do about food displays at the office, you can greatly reduce the temptation outside of it by avoiding restaurant lunches and dinners and by controlling the sea of food that seems to continuously wash up on your doorstep. Eat a light lunch at your desk and avoid buying unhealthy food, especially snacks like cookies and potato chips. Fill the refrigerator (at home and at work) with apples, oranges, grapes, strawberries, slices of melon, even a jar of carrot sticks in water. Replace the Oreos with a sweetened cereal like Cookie Crisp, which has much less fat and fewer calories. Still, keeping junk food out of your desk and out of your house are two different matters. If you have children, a house devoid of junk food is unrealistic—so avoid wherever you store them. If it's not mealtime, stay out of the kitchen.

But don't avoid the kitchen by settling into the den where the TV is. TV is your worst enemy. If all TV commercials consisted of deodorant soap dancing across the screen, it wouldn't be a problem. Unfortunately many commercials tempt you with food so tantalizing, you can almost taste and smell it. It's enough to launch you into an eating binge. When tormented by such temptation, your best recourse is to change the channel.

Curb Eating Momentum. Once a coworker complained to me that she felt hungrier after she ate than before. "Sometimes I wonder why I even bother to eat," she said. It's an old story: eating momentum unchecked by satiety. If you know this feeling, one tactic that will help you is to eat slower. This is no small order considering the hectic pace of today's living and the eat-and-go attitude of many executives. Yet it's important enough to affect how much you eat by a good margin. Gulping food leaves you prone to overeating because you finish in a flash and then sit at the table with nothing left to do but eat more, which you do, not stopping to notice that you've already had enough.

Another strategy is to wait for satiety. Satiety doesn't instantly kick in when the food hits your stomach. It could take as long as 20 minutes, while you hungrily scan the table for more food. But you know how much you've eaten, and it's usually enough, despite what your stomach is trying to tell you. Don't be tricked, be patient. Recognize that feeling hungry at times is a sign that you're achieving your goal of changing bad habits.

Eating on Business Travel Is No Different. Business travel is business as usual. Let that theme guide your eating. Whenever you travel on business, make it a goal to order what you would normally eat at home or at the office.

For example, what do you order for breakfast on the road? If it's eggs, sausage, hash browns, and biscuits, you need to go back to your reference, which is what you would eat at home. Would you eat such an elaborate breakfast at home? Not if you had to make it yourself, and certainly not if you want to improve your nutritional fitness. Hold the Eggs Benedict. Keep breakfasts eaten out simple and healthy. Order hot or cold cereal with fruit.

The same principle applies to lunch and dinner: eat as if you were at home. Many people order a cocktail at a business lunch or dinner, but they wouldn't dream of doing such a thing at home. Would you lead off a lunch at home with a glass of wine or a

Manhattan? Beer, wine, and liquor have no place in OptimEating. Loaded with empty calories—one gram of alcohol has seven calories, almost as much as fat—a cocktail or two can uninhibit you to the point that OptimEating doesn't seem necessary.

Remember, in the battle to control your weight, time is your ally. Use it to help gradually loosen the hold of fattening habits. In fact, use whatever tactics you can to replace your bad habits with good ones. They will lead you to your reward.

REWARD YOURSELF WITH YOUR FAVORITE FOOD

Only your reward pathway is capable of steering you toward new habits, of making it worth leaving old habits behind, of giving you enough reason to control your weight today and all the tomorrows that follow. The goal-reward circle discussed in Chapter 2, includes two kinds of rewards: intrinsic rewards that are internally generated by your reward pathway and extrinsic rewards that you give yourself. In weight control, goal accomplishment—specifically that of losing a number of pounds—is not a frequent enough intrinsic reward to fully support the effort required to change eating habits. No one should lose weight that fast, and no one can continue to lose it forever. Hence, the rewards in the third step of weight control are not intrinsic rewards but extrinsic rewards that are associated with behavior more than they are with goal achievement. This makes them more frequent.

But don't many of the reputable diets suggest extrinsic rewards? Yes, but the rewards they suggest don't work. Such rewards are misinterpretations of your needs, and they sabotage your weight-loss efforts.

Let's look at some popular rewards that vary in substance but are alike in their failure to control your weight. First, there are the transient rewards—new clothing, art objects, even vacations—that actually do stimulate your reward pathway. But how many new outfits can you buy? How many art objects can you collect? How many vacations can you go on? Not as many as your reward pathway needs to help you control your weight.

Then there are the unrealistic rewards that not only don't last, they never work to begin with. Many executives make the mistake of wishing for "if onlys." "If only I could lose weight": "I would get a promotion." "I would attract the opposite sex." "My spouse would treat me better." "I would be happy." But your losing weight won't manipulate the behavior of others or make you happy. "If only" rewards are never forthcoming, so you have no reason to change your eating habits.

Not even the reward of weight loss itself works. Say you set a realistic goal of losing 20 pounds in six months. After six months you've lost the weight and feel great. Do you continue to feel great? The answer is no. Of course you'll be pleased with your lower weight and svelte looks, but after a short time you'll take the "new you" for granted, and it will no longer be strong enough input for your reward pathway. Having been initially stimulated by the achievement of losing 20 pounds, your reward pathway is now hungry for more. But more it doesn't get, and without the proper stimulation it won't give you the feedback you desperately need. The pleasure that was holding you to new eating habits, giving you a reason to avoid fattening foods, is now gone.

Liquid diets program this failure. Designed to end abruptly, they stop the behavior that led to the weight loss. Again, without weight loss, your reward pathway is deprived of the goal achievement stimulation, and it leaves you asking yourself, "Is that all there is?" No, it isn't. There are steaks and pizzas and french fries and premium ice creams. What makes this scenario so inevitable is that the liquid diet never trained you to eat in the real world of food. No training and no support from your reward pathway—it's a setup for failure. In clinical terms this failure is called a relapse. But it's really a resumption of old behavior, the only behavior you know.

There is only one extrinsic reward that works in weight control—day after day, week after week, year after year: food. Food, above all other enticements, is a force in your life powerful enough to change you. What a paradox: the best and perhaps only way to change your eating habits is by rewarding yourself with the demon itself.

What better to look forward to than to eating your favorite food? And what comfort you'll feel knowing you won't have to give up the delicacies you love for the rest of your life. But you can't eat unlimited quantities of them. You must earn these rewards, and they must match your accomplishment.

How often should you reward yourself? If you have success-fully held off old habits during the day, don't celebrate with a dou-ble chocolate sundae at night. That just negates your success. A reasonable frequency is once a week—I prefer Sunday. I watch what I eat Monday through Saturday and reward myself on Sunday. It all depends on your goal and where you are in the OptimEating process—whether you're losing weight or whether you're main-taining it.

Because enjoyment is the core of the food reward's power, the reward should be the food you like the most. Here time is your ally. As time passes, the foods you previously took for granted or ate with intense guilt, will taste even better. It's as if eating them with-out self-hatred, which often accompanies chronic overeating of high-calorie foods, allows you to taste them more clearly, to enjoy them more intensely.

Watch for other changes too. As your habits change, so will your values: less will be enough. A special breakfast, for example, will no longer be two or three donuts, but one—that's all you'll want. A serving of cake, which used to weigh 6 ounces now only needs to weigh 3 ounces. Over time you'll find that less of a good thing will bring as much or greater enjoyment.

PLANNING FOR ENJOYMENT

Planning is the backbone of OptimEating. Unplanned or impromp-tu rewards weaken the tie between the special food and the behav-ior that earned it—if you had really earned it why didn't you plan it in the first place? No less important, it leaves you open to a binge. With a planned reward, you're more likely to follow the first two steps of OptimEating during a dinner out and then reward yourself at the end with a special dessert. But a last-minute decision, tinged with guilt, can easily explode into a martini, a chicken liver paté appetizer, a prime rib entree, followed, of course, by a chocolate soufflé dessert. Rationalizing rewards into binges may momentarily ease your conscience, but you can't kid your waistline.

Before you encounter any situation, decide in advance how you are going to handle it, even if the planning session occurs 5 minutes before the meal. Don't expect yourself to muster the necessary willpower while you're eating. Food can drive people to rationalize with creative powers they never knew they had and rationalizing is the antithesis of planning.

Plan ahead for a special occasion or celebration by "banking" negative calories—be a bit more strict about what you eat shortly before it. The celebration is an almost immediate reward for your efforts. Do not, however, execute this plan in reverse: indulge and cut back later. That turns OptimEating into a punishment. OptimEating is designed for reality. It recognizes that during holidays, vacations, or any other periods of celebration it's almost impossible not to gain a few pounds. Look at such weight gains as part of life, just as holidays and vacations are; not as a reason to lose confidence. By calmly resuming your OptimEating habits, you will drop that newly added weight.

Every day you must navigate an overflowing sea of notorious edibles that taste great but have a fat content that could launch your cholesterol level and your weight. This is a fact of life. What is a fact of sanity is that every so often you must be able to fish out of that sea some favorite delicacies. No real person should be expected to live without them. But the most generous reward system in the world won't ensure your OptimEating success if you don't have the right attitude. Your motive for eating should not be just to satiate your hunger, but to satiate it with a healthy, low-fat meal or snack.

Low-fat eating demands curiosity, creativity, experimentation, and a basic knowledge of nutrition. That's a lot to ask of even an executive, but compared to the rewards you'll receive—rewards that will be a lasting force in your life—it won't feel like a burden at all. In fact it will become fun.

As you maintain your OptimEating course, successfully avoiding fatty foods, your confidence will grow and you'll finally realize that you can control weight. What a victory. Revel in it and it will touch other areas of your life. If you can control your eating, you can control your temper. If you can keep weight off, you can climb higher on the corporate ladder. OptimEating is about success in general.

But remember that life is not an ongoing celebration; it's everyday living and eating punctuated by celebrations. Your job is to decide when those celebrations happen and what to do when they don't. At times this job will challenge you. But with OptimEating you'll meet the challenge. Twenty years ago I lost 50 pounds and finally kept it off. Yet my diet hasn't been static; it has changed constantly, building my confidence and improving my health. I am constantly planning for future enjoyment—anticipating my food reward for being a good eater. Whatever my circumstance is, I know I can control my weight.

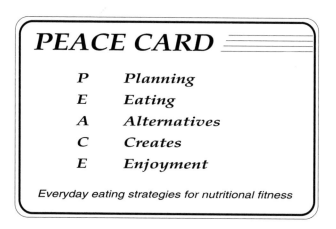

PEACE CARD

P	Planning
E	Eating
A	Alternatives
C	Creates
E	Enjoyment

Everyday eating strategies for nutritional fitness

CHAPTER 14

STRESS-ing RESILIENCY

Do you know what stress is? It's something every executive claims to have more than his share of—events, situations, encounters that descend upon you daily with the intent of destroying your peace of mind. Examples are plentiful: a peer "blind-sides" you by criticizing your work to your boss; an impossible deadline harasses you, and your key assistant is in the hospital; your company gives you the ultimatum of accepting a demotion or being laid off; your teenage daughter demands her own car; your spouse picked another fight with you. You know what stress is.

But do you really? If you were financially strapped and were told that your car needed $600 dollars of transmission work, you would view the news as stress. Would it be stressful if you had ample money to buy a new car? No. What's at work here is more than just a stressful event; it's how the event affects you. The vague villain stress is really two distinct things: the stressor and the stress response.

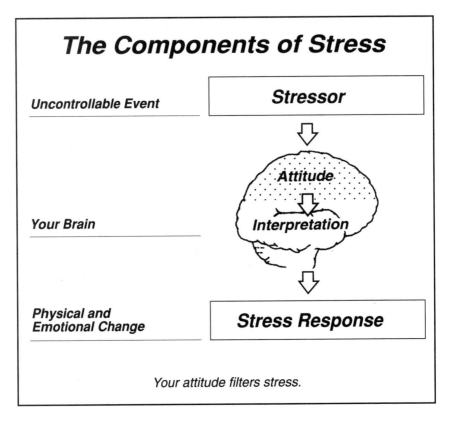

The Components of Stress

Uncontrollable Event	**Stressor**

Attitude

Interpretation

Physical and Emotional Change	***Stress Response***

Your attitude filters stress.

STRESS IS IN THE MIND OF THE BEHOLDER

The *stressor* is an event, usually external—your teenage daughter's unreasonable demand, the broken car transmission—over which you usually have no control. The greater your exposure to uncontrollable events, the greater your exposure to stressors. Such exposure is part of being an executive. Less common are the internal stressors, such as illness and injury. But in all cases the stressor is an event, and that's all.

What you feel when confronted with a stressor is your *stress response*. YOU, and only you, have the ability to empower a stressor by interpreting it in such a way that it upsets you. How you view the broken transmission is what's important. Stress is in the mind of the beholder.

One person's stressor is another person's pleasure. As an emergency room doctor, I wanted patients to come in; it gave my students the opportunity to help real people, instead of reading about how to do it in a textbook. But a colleague of mine saw an influx of patients differently. He found a busy emergency room intolerable and fled to the coffee shop when things heated up. We were both subjected to the same stressor, yet his anxiety and blood pressure were far different than mine. Our stress responses were opposite.

A negative stress response can seriously damage your physical and emotional health. In humankind's evolution the stress response was nature's way of dealing with life-threatening situations. It summoned a broad range of physical and emotional changes: fear, anger, and anxiety; quickened pulse and raised blood pressure; neurological, hormonal, and circulatory changes—all meant to prepare a human to take a stand or run for his life. In medicine we call this the fight or flight response.

Today, of course, humans must still cope with real danger. But real danger is not the stressor so many people who routinely generate the fight or flight response react to. They walk around in a continuous state of alarm over an argument with a coworker, or over a negative turn in the stock market, or over an impending corporate reorganization, or over the fear that they are going to lose their job. Not that losing your job is a small matter. It is a bona fide crisis. Nevertheless, high blood pressure and all the other unhealthy responses, including a suppressed immune system, do nothing to help the situation—in fact, they impair your ability to cope with it.

Even worse, negative physical responses feed negative emotional responses, which in turn, feed more negative physical responses. It's a wicked cycle brought on by the brain's habit of monitoring the body. Unchecked, this cycle whirls into a chronic stress response. In today's corporate environment inappropriate stress responses seem to be the rule, not the exception.

Living by such a rule, you are far more vulnerable to other stressors. Now something that wouldn't have upset you before is capable of triggering a full-blown stress response. Some people caught in this cycle don't even know how to get out of it, and some don't even know that they are in it. It has become a way of life. But a life of being drained physically and emotionally is *not* a life of being fit.

No one can remove all the stressors from his life. But you can learn to control your stress responses by building stress resilience in much the same way you build cardio or muscular fitness—with a program.

SHAPING YOUR ATTITUDE

Like cardio endurance and muscular fitness, nutritional health and stress resilience, attitude is a component of total fitness. But it is a special component because it is a precursor to all the other components. You'll never achieve good nutrition or cardio fitness if you don't have the right attitude. And it has the most influence on stress resilience.

Your attitude is the prevailing way you look at the world, the filter through which all stressors must pass before they are evaluated by your psyche. This is a strategic position. As the first barrier that stress meets, attitude has a magnifying effect, and a small change in it has a large effect on the stress response. Therefore, your first step toward stress resilience is to change your attitude. Adopt characteristics of a fit attitude and discard those of an unfit one.

Figure 14.1 is a list of traits found in fit and unfit attitudes. No one has a totally fit or unfit attitude—we all have our good and bad points. It is the dominance of good traits overruling the bad ones that forms a fit attitude, or the dominance of bad ones that poison it. A bad attitude is a deadly poison. How many times have you heard someone say, "He has a lousy attitude"? Unfortunately, he probably has much more than a lousy attitude. From an unfit attitude come many physical and emotional problems. Pat is a good example of this. An attorney who was both impatient and hostile, she constantly finds fault with the people around her. Her secretary never works fast enough and "purposely" refused to learn the billing system. Her boss is always dumping his case load on her. "He's been on the phone all day planning his vacation in Europe," she once complained. Every day it is something else. With an attitude like that it's no surprise that Pat suffers from back problems and migraine headaches, and with bizarre frequency "catches" someone else's "stomach virus." None of Pat's problems are life

Figure 14.1	ATTITUDE CHARACTERISTICS

Fit	Unfit
Optimistic – Positive	Pessimistic – Negative
Caring – Warm	Isolated – Cold
Calm – Relaxed	Tense – Anxious
Accepting – Patient	Blaming – Complaining
Accommodating – Flexible	Perfectionist – Rigid
Helpfulness – Supportive	Aggressive – Controlling
Humorous – Jovial	Anger – Hostility
Empathetic – Understanding	Superior – Aloof
Persistent – Deliberate	Impatient – Impulsive

threatening, but her future is ominous. Ailments also related to unfit traits are cancer, heart disease, and rheumatoid arthritis, to name just a few.

A fit attitude has the opposite effect, bolstering the immune system and slashing the probability of succumbing to emotional problems. Ray, a director of systems, never seemed to be in a bad mood—probably because he never let anything rankle him. One day after commuting to work in an unheated train he remarked, "You could see your breath on that train. It was another frosty ride." The remark wasn't angry—in fact it was cheerful. I don't remember Ray ever being sick. Both the body and the mind need a fit attitude. To have one, if only sporadically, is to be healthier.

Looking at the list of traits, you may feel uneasy, remembering how angry and impatient you got when your flight home was canceled. A distinction should therefore be made between what qualifies as an angry and impatient attitude and what doesn't. In some situations only a saint can remain calm. But an angry and impatient person is someone who seethes whenever the slightest thing doesn't go his way. Usually this person is also pessimistic and negative; he expects problems and he gets them.

At the other extreme, you may not recognize any unfit traits in yourself; they have become so deeply ingrained in your thinking that you don't think you have a problem. What you think is that the problem is "out there," not in here. If that's how you feel, get a reality check from "out there." Ask people you trust how they see you. Are you a pessimist? Do you get angry too easily? Do you come on too strongly? Are you a perfectionist? You may get some eye-opening replies. Evaluate them honestly and accept them positively by looking forward to the pleasant experiences that adjusting your attitude can create.

After you've thoroughly examined your inner self, you can work on shaping your attitude into what you want it to be. At times you will have to act one way even when you feel another. This takes effort, but it's more effective than just trying *not* to act a certain way. When you say you are *not* going to be impatient, half of your brain doesn't recognize the *not,* hearing instead "I am going to be impatient." The result is confusion, and a confused brain won't change you. Bad attitudes don't evaporate when you tell them to get lost. They get replaced by good attitudes.

This takes persistence and a deep desire to change. Sometimes an unfit trait like anger will be hard to give up, especially if you feel it is justified. But anger—justified or not—is unhealthy. The question is: how do you stop this trait from controlling you? Start by acting calm and constructive while reminding yourself how damaging it is to be angry. Do this consistently, and you will begin to notice that you don't get so easily angered anymore. Or you may feel justified in blaming someone for something. In that case, take the opposite approach by trying to explain their point of view. This will not only weaken the habit of blaming, it will diffuse the anger that so often accompanies it.

But don't wait until you are confronted with an irritating situation to apply the technique of attitude shaping. Rehearse the correct response throughout the day. First, write on a cue card how you want to act in specific situations, one situation per card. These cards will be your new script. Then read the cards several times a day, amending them with some self-talk to enhance your performance. Strive for an Oscar®.

Your Inner Judge's Role in Interpreting Stressors

But no one's attitude can be shaped perfectly enough to filter out every stressor in his or her life. What happens to a stressor that gets through your attitude filter depends on your interpretation of it. Lurking somewhere between your conscious and subconscious is a judgmental interpreter. I call this interpreter the Hanging Judge—and for good reason. Here is where your criticism of yourself and others is born, where the script that blames and complains is written, where catastrophizing an event is justified, where the color of negativity that so thickly coats life is painted. When this judge is allowed to interpret a stressor, it presses all panic buttons, and then berates you for not handling it flawlessly.

We all have a Hanging Judge. What differs is the power it has over our individual lives; some people's judges are more powerful than other people's. Initially, your Hanging Judge was created to give you much needed guidance during your childhood. But as an adult, you don't need it anymore. It should have been impeached long ago. Yet rarely does this happen. Instead, it is permitted to sit on the bench throughout your adulthood and wield its destructive power. One way it survives is by cleverness: it has so integrated itself into your thought process that you aren't aware of its presence, just feelings of anxiety, anger or depression. Those feelings are red warning lights. So are such statements as "I must." "I can't." "Now look what you've done." "This is the worst thing that could have happened." When you feel anxious, angry or depressed, or hear yourself saying that kind of thing, recognize that your Hanging Judge is clamoring for a harsh sentence and offering you no mercy—as usual.

Criticizing, a favorite activity of the Hanging Judge, rarely adds anything positive to a situation and frequently pummels the person who does it. Those who are critical of others tend to be even more critical of themselves. Counter this habit by replacing your standard critical comments about other people with harmless statements such as, "Let's pull together on this" or "That's another way to look at it"—any statement that's empathetic. Use the same statement for all situations and people, including yourself. Don't let your Hanging Judge have the last word. Talk over him—shout if necessary—dare to be in contempt of court. Before long you'll notice that you're less critical of everything.

Another common activity of your Hanging Judge is *blaming* problems on someone else. You blame them; then you complain about them. It seems so easy: just dump the onus elsewhere. But what you think lightens the load of responsibility only angers you and distorts the truth. Like an irritating recording, the blaming and complaining play over and over, sapping your energy. If fault is to be found, find it, let it go, and move on. Leave your judge without a case to try.

Your Hanging Judge, however, will not give up its power without a struggle; it has other sabotage in store for you. It thrives on your predicting a horrible ending to a crisis or problem. *Catastrophizing,* as this is called, often starts when you become pre-occupied with the impact of a stressor on your future. John, a 35-year-old personnel manager at an electronics company, lost his job in a corporate-wide cutback. Living in a small town, he knew he couldn't find another comparable job there; he would have to relo-cate. With that realization, his world crumbled. "I'll never be able to sell my house," he said. "If I can't sell my house, I can't relocate for another job. I'll end up in debt—forever. My children will hate me." A year later, John was anxious, depressed, and still out of work. At that point, his children probably did resent him. Catastrophizing didn't help him through a crisis, nor will it help you. It only distracts by inciting fear, anger, anxiety, and depression.

Whenever you are confronted with a crisis, don't let your Hanging Judge hear the case. Calmly talk to yourself as you would to a close friend who is so emotionally wrapped up in a crisis he can't think clearly. What would you say to calm him down? Often when people remove themselves from the emotional tangle of a cri-sis, they can think more clearly. The more you reason with your inner "friend," questioning his dark logic and pointing out positive approaches, the better you feel. Do this for minor problems as well as major crises. Polish this technique with practice, and your inner "friend" will become much more stress resilient.

Recognizing Your Stress Responses

Stressors are relatively easy to recognize—they are events, they happen. But how do you know whether your attitude successfully filters the stressor or, if not, that your interpretation of it is toxic? How do you know if you're having a stress response?

Like most people, you probably walk around in the throes of a moderate stress response marked by vague feelings of anxiety, or jumpiness and irritability, or muscular tension, or many other physical or emotional symptoms, even though they are not at a fever pitch. These miseries you live with continuously. You don't even recognize they're present until they become magnified by a real stressor. To you they are "normal." But it's an unhealthy normal. A continuous stress response batters your body and mind.

If "normal" is unhealthy, what then is a healthy, stress-free state? A good way to answer that is to imagine how you feel right before you take off on a week of vacation. Compare that to the way you feel now (unless you're on vacation). There is probably a very big difference. But why should there be? Is there, in reality, such a big difference between your life before a week of vacation and a week of work? No. Yet how differently you feel. It's a difference that demonstrates the negative power an ongoing stress response has over your life.

Another way to detect a stress response is to ask yourself these questions: "Do I have difficulty concentrating or coming up with creative ideas?" "Am I less decisive than I want to be or than I have been before?" "Do I feel on edge or irritable most of the time?" "Have I lost my ability to enjoy things I used to?" "Is my list of outside interests shrinking?" Though these questions highlight some mental symptoms of a chronic stress response, the physical symptoms are no less distressing. Headaches, back pain—in fact, almost any ache or pain—even inflamed joints can be traced to stress.

The kind of stressors that cause stress responses differ for everyone. Sometimes it's not just one noticeable stressor but many little ones. The misplaced sales report, the cocktail reception you'd rather not go to, the lost car keys, the discovery that there is no milk in the house, the leaking faucet, each a minor stressor that won't cause a stress response until it is combined with another stressor.

Watch for small stressors too. Take them one by one and talk to your inner "friend" about them. Point out how small each is and why it shouldn't bother him. Tell him why he should feel better—and you will.

Stressors and our stress responses to them aren't always obvious. In many cases they go unnoticed; people accept them as part of life. Well that's not living; it's surviving—if that. Strengthen your stress resilience and feel good for a change.

AVOID SELF-INFLICTED STRESS

You can improve your stress resilience in many ways. I've already explained that shaping your attitude with positive characteristics will filter a great many stressors. Other fitness components that affect stress are nutrition and cardio exercise. Eating nutritiously, instead of skipping meals and eating too many sugary snacks, will strengthen your resilience. And aerobic exercise has been proven to produce positive, happy thoughts in runners, even if they were anxious or depressed before their run.

Later, I will describe some "exercises" you can do that were specifically designed to improve stress resilience. But first, you should know about four common aspects of executive life that can significantly affect your stress response.

Beware of Caffeine Addiction

Coffee happens to be the most common addiction found in executives. Not that the coffee itself is to blame; it's the caffeine it contains that causes the problem. Caffeine is physically and psychologically addictive in the same way that heroin is, but not nearly as powerful in its grip. Nevertheless, a caffeine addiction is powerful enough to increase your tension and anxiety. Valium, a drug frequently used to treat stress responses, relieves a person's anxiety by activating a certain receptor in the brain. Caffeine *blocks* that same receptor. Drinking over five cups of coffee a day, you wash away some of your stress resilience because of what caffeine does in the brain. In other words, coffee becomes a stressor itself.

In the arena of business, where executives are so constantly pounded by stressors over which they have no control, it's tragic that so many of them weaken themselves with something they can control—their coffee drinking. If you drink over five cups a day, cut down to three. But do it slowly. Sudden withdrawal from caffeine bombards you with a brutal headache and slows you physically and mentally. Stretch your usual time intervals between cups by substituting decaffeinated for regular. The decaffeinated coffee creates an illusion of having the real thing: it looks the same, tastes the same, and smells the same, there in your cup in its usual spot on your desk. Illusion goes a long way.

Of course there will be times when you feel tired, and you want an extra cup of coffee for a little push. That's all right as long as it doesn't become a habit and escalate from there. (See Figure 14.2 for familiar products that contain caffeine.)

Figure 14.2 PRODUCTS CONTAINING CAFFEINE

Product	Caffeine (mg)	Product	Caffeine (mg)
Coffee		**Soft Drinks**	
Drip or perk (6 oz)	80–180	Coke (12 oz)	45
Instant (6 oz)	50–130	Pepsi (12 oz)	35
Dunkin Donuts (8 oz)	100	Mountain Dew (12 oz)	55
McDonald's (6 oz)	80	Mellow Yellow (12 oz)	40
Starbucks (6 oz)	80	Dr Pepper (12 oz)	40
Gloria Jeans (6.4 oz)	80	Mr Pibb (12 oz)	40
Coffee Beanery (8 oz)	100	RC (12 oz)	40
Au Bon Pain (9 oz)	171	Sun Bolt (12 oz)	40
Decaffeinated (6 oz)	2–6	Big Red Cola (12 oz)	40
Espresso		**Medications**	
Au Bon Pain (2.5 oz)	130	Anacin (2 tablets)	64
Gloria Jeans (2.7 oz)	51	Excedrin (2 tablets)	130
Coffee Beanery (2.4 oz)	84	Empirin (2 tablets)	64
Capuccino		Midol (2 tablets)	64
Specialty shop (8 oz)	50–80	Vanquish (2 tablets)	64
Instant (8 oz)	35–115	**Other**	
Tea		Coffee-flavored yogurt (8 oz)	45
Steeped 3 minutes (6 oz)	20–50	Bittersweet chocolate (1 oz)	5–35
Steeped 5 minutes (6 oz)	50–100	Cadbury chocolate (1 oz)	15

The Truth About Alcohol

Many executives wrestle with another addiction—alcoholism. Far more devastating than coffee, alcohol is used not to boost a person, but to soothe him, to help him escape from the bombardment of stressors and the tyranny of his stress response.

Alcoholism usually sneaks up on the executive. At first the problem isn't obvious to the victim or his co-workers (see Figure 14.3); the impairment it causes is minor, though certainly not negligible, and his talent and intelligence make up for it. He continues to get a "fix" easily; business lunches, dinners, and cocktail hours all give him the opportunity to drink. But the party doesn't last forever. "Executive" alcoholism is marked by a daily need for alcohol that increases through the years, and eventually its stunting effect on personal and professional growth begins to surface. Now the executive needs alcohol to function.

Figure 14.3 **CLUES TO ALCOHOL VULNERABILITY**

---

1. A close relative who is an alcoholic.

2. The ability to drink more than the average person without feeling or manifesting the effects.

3. More than the equivalent of two drinks (1 ounce each) of alcohol per day.

4. A conviction for driving while impaired or intoxicated.

5. Looking forward to, planning, and manipulating alcohol consumption on a daily basis.

6. Drinking before 11:00 A.M.

7. An unsuccessful attempt to decrease intake.

8. Shakiness, difficulty concentrating, or anxiety relieved by alcohol.

9. Friends or relatives *telling* you that you have a problem.

10. You drink more on a regular basis than you did five years ago.

This is the most diabolical tragedy of all. He can't function with it and he can't function without it. Further compounding the matter is the fact that alcohol is toxic. As the problem outgrows the acceptable boundaries of social drinking, it dulls the mind and depletes the body. Alcohol has become a major stressor. No executive can function under this oppression.

Eventually, everyone notices the problem—that is, everyone except the executive—but his position in the company and community may prevent them from approaching him about it. This is a tragedy. Only when the alcoholic recognizes his problem will he be able to cure it.

Withdrawing from alcohol is not easy. The measures the alcoholic must take depend on the severity of the problem. Most alcoholics need the support of their family and friends, of their company and of support groups like Alcoholics Anonymous. Whatever course an alcoholic chooses, education on the topic is a must—newsletters, clinical studies, testimonials.

The nondrinking executive used to stand out like an oddball. Fifteen years ago a senior accountant in an international public accounting firm told me that a staff member was expected to order a drink when out to lunch with a client—as if drinking was part of some professional code of behavior. Whether top management really felt that way was not important. Most of the professional staff thought that management did. Today the nondrinking executive stands out as a healthier, stronger professional. Maybe it's because businesses are beginning to recognize alcohol's impact on their bottom line. Alcohol is a deadly stressor.

Sleeping Problems

Yet everyone "knows" that alcohol relaxes you and helps you sleep. Surely if you need a good night's sleep, especially when traveling, a nightcap can't do any harm.

But it can. Alcohol disrupts your sleep. True, it helps you fall asleep, but falling asleep and sleeping well are two different matters. Sleep consists of different cycles. Disrupt these cycles—with alcohol or any other substance—and you downgrade the quality of your sleep. Poor quality sleep, in turn, downgrades your stress resilience.

Most people don't link sleep problems with weakened stress resilience; they link it to feeling lousy. But what does feeling lousy mean? It means you can't concentrate or solve problems or make decisions. It means you can't handle a stressor as effectively; you are too busy trying to marshall your personal assets, your mind and body, to meet it. It means that a dark haze has settled over you.

This dark haze is a stressor itself, but unlike many stressors, it's one you can control. Disperse it by improving the quality of your sleep. Alcohol isn't the only sleep disrupter. Examine your habits. Do you consume caffeine after 6:00 P.M.? Avoid anything that contains caffeine—coffee, soft drinks, analgesics. Do your bedtimes vary during the week? Establish regular bedtime habits: go to bed the same time every night and get up the same time every morning. Do you watch the 11:00 P.M. news? Find out what's going on in the world before 7:00 P.M.; then go to bed with a peaceful mind and wake up early enough to exercise.

Dealing with Jet Lag

Many businesses operate coast to coast, country to country. Obviously, crossing borders complicates matters: cultural and currency differences must be accounted for. But executives have learned to deal with these factors. What executives haven't learned to deal with is jet lag.

Not that business travelers haven't tried. A few years ago some people took valium-like medications to help them sleep during long flights so they would be well rested and thus less vulnerable to jet lag. It seemed to work until the next day. Then the troubled traveler suffered from periods of amnesia and impaired reasoning ability—not a good way to do business.

Today, business travelers are at it again, looking to a pop-in-your-mouth cure for a common malady. This time it's the hormone melatonin. Sold over-the-counter, melatonin supplements are not regulated; there is no way to tell what other substances they contain, such as impurities, and impurities were the downfall of L-tryptophan, the amino acid in vogue a few years back as a treatment for insomnia and depression. But the most important reason not to take melatonin is that it's a powerful hormone that affects the human body in ways not completely understood. The body's feedback mechanism is extremely complex, involving hormones other than melatonin and systems other than its biological clock. It's pure speculation that melatonin cures jet lag. Is speculation reason enough to play pharmacological games with your brain's hormone levels?

Following are some safer, and proven, tactics to help you adjust to changing time zones:

1. Avoid alcohol; it aggravates jet lag.

2. Avoid medications with sedative side effects, such as allergy and cold remedies.

3. Eat lightly; heavy, fatty meals tend to decrease concentration, which is already impaired by jet lag.

4. Exercise (aerobically) in the morning to help you sleep better.

5. Within reason, continue to wake up and fall asleep on home time rather than local time.

Exercises to Improve Your Stress Resilience

A fit attitude and a lifestyle of good eating, of quality sleeping, and of exercising should build an excellent stress resilience. Still, lifelong reactions to stress aren't easily changed. To help you move toward your goal, I've included five exercises. Practice these to become adept at doing them. Then use them routinely or as needed whenever stress strikes.

Abdominal Breathing. Abdominal breathing is easy to learn but difficult to do continuously. Most people breathe in a shallow, erratic pattern of inhaling and exhaling, and to steady the pattern, to inhale deeper, would at first require almost constant attention to their breathing. This is no small effort. Still, abdominal breathing is a good way to control a stress response, even if you do it only when you're troubled.

When you breathe abdominally, you get more air into your lungs with much less effort. Athletes, of course, love this.

Conserving energy contributes to their chances of winning. Elite endurance runners, for example, breathe abdominally when they race, but for more than extra energy: abdominal breathing promotes relaxation—another performance enhancer. For you, abdominal breathing can calm a severe physical or emotional stress response. That's what I call performance enhancing.

The technique is simple. Begin by taking a slow full deep breath and then letting it out slowly. On your second inhalation expand your stomach as if you are filling it with air. The inhalation and exhalation—done slowly, deliberately, and rhythmically—should take equal amounts of time. Initially this may feel uncomfortable because it is so different from the regular way you breathe but that is short-lived; what calms you quickly becomes comfortable. Practice makes better (not perfect), and the better you get at abdominal breathing, the more effectively it will reduce your level of tension—whether or not you are under the gun.

LOOSEN UP AND RELAX. Many people have nervous habits that are part of their behavior every day, and unless it's smoking, they'll probably tell you it's harmless. Alan, the assistant controller of a multinational manufacturing company, thought his habits were harmless. One of those habits I'll call tape rolling. During meetings in his office, Alan would grab a tape dispenser, tear off a small piece of tape, attach its ends so it formed a circle, and stick and unstick his thumb and index finger to it repeatedly. Alan had a whole battery of nervous habits. Even his laugh was high pitched and nervous—as if he pushed it out of his throat.

What Alan didn't realize or wouldn't admit was that his nervous habits escalated, becoming more numerous, more frantic, especially during year-end closings, and that they were increasing his overall body tension. He was trapped in a vicious cycle. A basic tenet of human behavior is that a fidgety habit makes you *feel* anxious, which in turn makes you more fidgety. Therefore remain as quiet and as calm as you can. Try not to bounce your leg, tap your fingers, or squeeze your forehead. Don't move hastily, speak rapidly (another of Alan's habits), or hold a rigid posture. These physical habits feed tension. The brain picks them up and wonders what's wrong, and if it's not obvious, it will find something. That's when your muscles start to get tenser and tenser. Constant muscular tension can lead to back and jawbone problems. So be more fluid in your movements, walk with a relaxed gait—even if you're in a rush—and practice relaxing.

One way to relax is by progressive relaxation. (See Figure 14.4.) I break this procedure into two steps. Step 1 consists of consciously tensing up your entire body to the point of muscle fatigue, then releasing the tension. In step 2 you again tense and relax, but only one part of the body at a time until you have covered your entire body; for example, your feet first, then your legs, torso, and so on. If time is short, try what I call target calming. First note what muscles are tight. Then focus on relaxing just those muscles. This is particularly good for the notorious strongholds of bodily tension, the upper and lower back and the jaw and the front temples, which when relaxed induce a decrease in the entire body's tension. Another shortcut is to relax your muscles without first tensing them. Try this after you've practiced the tensing kind; only then can you tell if it's just as effective. Neither progressive relaxation nor target calming take much time. But the deep muscle relaxation they bring feels both physically and emotionally wonderful.

INTROSPECTIVE MEDITATION. Introspective meditation is a simple technique that requires no formal training. When most people think of meditation, they picture someone sitting cross-legged, chanting a mantra, and to a certain extent this meditation is similar. You can do it sitting cross-legged, chanting a mantra. But you can also do it lying down, or sitting against a wall with your legs outstretched in front of you or in any position that keeps your head, neck and spine in a straight line. I do it sitting because I fall asleep when lying down. Whatever position you choose, you must quiet your mind by concentrating on one of three things.

1. *Create a picture in your mind's eye.* It can be a candle's flame or a leaf floating down a stream or a field being silently covered by snowflakes—any scene you find peaceful and calming.

2. *Repeat a word or phrase over and over.* Also called a mantra, it should suggest peacefulness or calmness or contentment. "Peace," "Calm," "God is with me" are all examples, but the best mantra is what's meaningful to you.

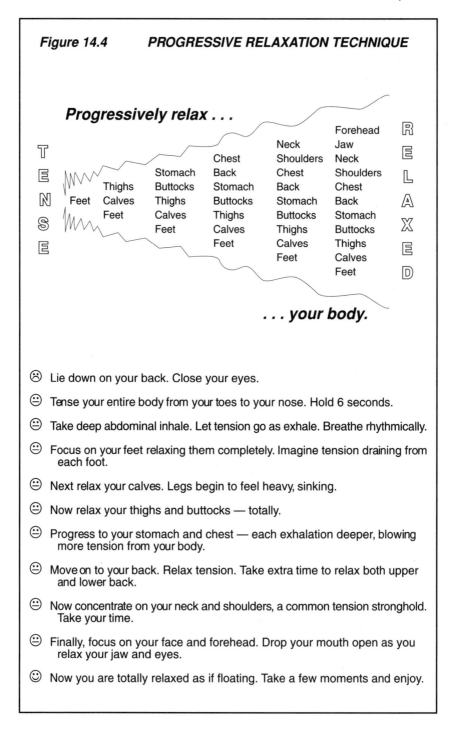

Figure 14.4 *PROGRESSIVE RELAXATION TECHNIQUE*

Progressively relax . . .

. . . **your body.**

☹ Lie down on your back. Close your eyes.

☺ Tense your entire body from your toes to your nose. Hold 6 seconds.

☺ Take deep abdominal inhale. Let tension go as exhale. Breathe rhythmically.

☺ Focus on your feet relaxing them completely. Imagine tension draining from each foot.

☺ Next relax your calves. Legs begin to feel heavy, sinking.

☺ Now relax your thighs and buttocks — totally.

☺ Progress to your stomach and chest — each exhalation deeper, blowing more tension from your body.

☺ Move on to your back. Relax tension. Take extra time to relax both upper and lower back.

☺ Now concentrate on your neck and shoulders, a common tension stronghold. Take your time.

☺ Finally, focus on your face and forehead. Drop your mouth open as you relax your jaw and eyes.

☺ Now you are totally relaxed as if floating. Take a few moments and enjoy.

3. *Listen to each breath as you draw it in and let it out.* Inhale and exhale through your nose. Ideally this should be abdominal breathing.

At first your mind may not be easily quieted—other thoughts such as planning or worrying may smother your candle flame or drown out your mantra or breathing. This is not unusual. Simply let the thoughts go without becoming upset over their intrusion, and return to your point of concentration. Sometimes it's helpful to act like a detached spectator. Separate yourself from your thoughts, calmly watching them leave as if they have nothing to do with you.

I recommend meditating daily for 10 to 20 minutes. But you don't need to do it for that long or even regularly to reap some benefits; impromptu sessions are also helpful. Helen, a manager of consolidations at a pharmaceutical company, had been meditating daily for three months. "My meditating time was right after I got home from work," she said. Then year-end came. "I started working late and couldn't meditate as often." But when Helen was given a special project in the middle of that busy time, she started meditating on the job. "I was seething," she said. "They [top management] just don't know all the work that goes into putting these numbers together. At that point I knew I needed to take a time-out or I wasn't going to get any work done. So I found an empty conference room and meditated for five minutes." Afterward Helen returned to her office and calmly continued to work. It had made a big difference. "At least I knew I'd done the right thing," she said. Just find a quiet spot, ask not to be disturbed, and meditate.

SOFT EYES. Frequently, a tense person will become hypervigilant; their eyes take on a darting, piercing quality that most people have come to expect from a high-powered executive. But this is not a healthy way to look at things. The face is a very sensitive mirror of an individual's emotions—so sensitive that depression can be diagnosed simply by measuring the face's muscular activity. Far more sensitive is the brain's monitoring system. Again we see the physical state leading the mental one. The brain constantly scans the body's muscular tension—especially the facial tension—and makes assumptions based on its readings. If it reads that the muscles around the eyes are showing the tension patterns of a vigilant state, it will then boost the emotional and physical tension throughout the body. Escalating tension is unhealthy, yet people walk around with their eyes darting vigilantly all the time.

Unlike darting, restless eyes, soft eyes maintain a calm, restful look. From the inside looking out, soft eyes see with clear vision, yet they don't focus on anything in particular. A person with a soft outlook tells his brain there is nothing to worry about, and his brain, believing it, decreases the intensity of the stress response.

STAY IN THE PRESENT. A great number of your inappropriate stress responses stem from dwelling on past failures or worrying about their negative impact on the future. By doing this you ignore the present, otherwise known as reality. It requires far less thought to deal with the present than it does to hash over the seemingly endless negative possibilities of the future. But many people have spent their lives *out* of the present, and living *in* it is something they must learn to do.

This will take some effort. Remind yourself to stay in the present by putting a note card on your desk. It can read "stay in the present" or "pay attention"—anything that jolts your thoughts back to where they belong. George's thoughts were far from there when he was returning from vacation to a dreadful work situation. Walking around the airport, he wondered how much work was piled on his desk, what the consultants' report would say, whether he would be able to replace the assistant buyer who was leaving. "I was absolutely miserable," he said, "thinking of one work disaster after another." What spared George from his own thought torture was his realization that he was a thousand miles from his office, and that there was nothing he could do about the work piled on his desk or the consultants breathing down his neck. "To pry my mind away from those worries," he said, "I started to look around me and notice what was going on. I saw a young man in the Navy and wondered why he enlisted in that branch of the military. I saw a family walking by and wondered where they lived." That was George's refuge. He walked around noticing things and asking himself questions about them. None of the questions did he need to answer. The point is that they were occupying his mind instead of his worries. "It wasn't long before that awful feeling was gone," he said.

Whenever your mind is full of worries, or you're in the grip of a full-blown stress response, step back from the turmoil and quietly observe what's going on around you. Watch raindrops striking your window, leaves falling, or people walking on the street. Ask questions as George did. Even supply your own answers. Crowd out of your mind all that you *can't* do anything about at that moment. Be at peace.

Of all the components of fitness, stress resilience is the one that is more relevant to the executive than it is to the general population. Give stress resilience the attention it deserves. Set a goal to rid yourself of unhealthy stress responses. When you design a program, include stress exercises along with your aerobic and anaerobic ones. No executive fitness program, whether it belongs to a man or a woman, is complete without it.

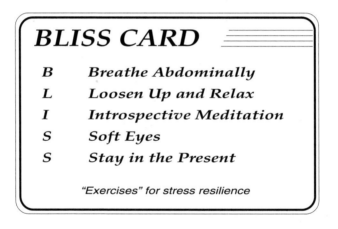

BLISS CARD	
B	**Breathe Abdominally**
L	**Loosen Up and Relax**
I	**Introspective Meditation**
S	**Soft Eyes**
S	**Stay in the Present**

"Exercises" for stress resilience

· CHAPTER 15 ·

A MAN'S PROGRAM

Five years ago Greg, a nurse at the hospital where I worked, approached me with news about his personal health breakthrough. "Doctor Pace," he said, "I've been taking 325 milligrams of iron a day for over a year now and I feel great." I was shocked. Even Greg, a health care professional, had been misinformed and was taking a dose of iron that was good for anemic patients but potentially harmful for him. My response: "Stop taking the iron." Unlike women, men rarely need iron supplementation.

For today's executive, many fitness issues—diet, exercise, stress management—are getting whipped in the blender of sexual equality and poured into one, big unisex glass. As a response to equality issues, it represents little improvement over the past for the male executive. Most fitness programs of the past were designed for men, with much emphasis placed on aerobic or anaerobic exercise. Now eating, stress management, and flexibility—health concerns no fitness program should be without—are included, but only as vague generalities gleaned from both sexes. Unfortunately, generalities fit neither men nor women. They misinform them, as in Greg's case.

The most effective fitness program must be designed for one sex. First, there are obvious psychological differences that stem from different cultural input and variations in the brain's organization itself. And no two men are alike either. Though physiologically similar, men can have pronounced differences in skeletal structure and muscle development, not to mention contrasting psychological outlooks. All this points out that every man needs the knowledge to design his own fitness program.

"A Man's Program" discusses each component of fitness in the order of its probable importance. That order may not apply to you. Nutrition, for example, may be more important than cardio because you already exercise aerobically, or stress may be more important while you go through a difficult period. Whatever component you start with, it should be the one most lacking in your life.

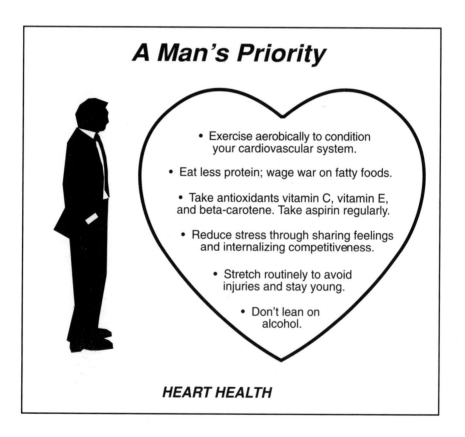

Aerobic Conditioning for the Heart

The number one priority for men is to prevent heart disease. Unlike women, whose hormones protect their hearts until menopause, men must mount a defense as young adults. Long before the male's number one killer takes his life, it robs him of his vigor and productivity. While this physical deterioration is reluctantly accepted by the average man who eyes retirement to salvage what's left of his life, the executive is cut down in his prime. Having amassed the experience and knowledge necessary to ascend in his profession, he now finds his new limits governed by medications and fatigue. This tragedy is entirely avoidable.

Therefore, go sweat, young men—and older men too. Your first line of defense is aerobic exercise. What kind of aerobic exercise doesn't matter as long as it keeps your heart pumping hard enough. This is consistent with a man's concept of exercise, which is synonymous with a vigorous workout. Not so with a woman. Put through a strenuous workout, she is more likely to abandon it, preferring instead to exercise less intensely. Is this an advantage? Does a man's favoring a vigorous workout improve his odds of becoming a long-term exerciser? Recent history says no.

If you push your heart rate into the heart-healthy range of 60 to 75 percent of your pulse limit, before your heart has been conditioned, before your muscles have developed endurance, you will suffer during and after the workout. This might feed the "no pain, no gain" mind-set of some men who mistake pain as their goal, but it will not drive an executive. Your downfall is in your dedication to any commitment you undertake. The pain is something you accept stoically, dues you must pay to become fit. But this dedication disappears when the first injury strikes. Wounded by this supposedly healthy activity, you understandably feel betrayed.

Injuries are the number one reason men give up exercising. But this statistic is misleading. It suggests that injuries are a fact of exercise, when they are really the result of mistakes. Yet knowing that exercise should be adopted gradually does not alter the outcome for many executives. They merely apply the tried and true risk-taking approach that so competently moved them up the corporate ladder. But risk taking in the business environment is a means of strengthening and expanding the company in the face of fierce competition, and ultimately it translates into rewards for the executive—raises, promotions, and other fringe benefits. That is not the case with your personal fitness. The risk of pushing yourself harder and longer will not reward you; it will undermine your exercise program with injuries. Injuries are inconvenient, painful, and expensive. It's no wonder that so many exercise programs file for bankruptcy.

The message here is loud and clear: when you begin an exercise program, work out at intensities *below* the heart-healthy range, moving into its low end—60 percent of your pulse limit (see Figure 15.1)—only after you have preconditioned your muscles. There you can get a vigorous workout without drowning in your own sweat, and there you can stay for the rest of your life. In conditioning the heart, the law of diminishing returns applies; it won't get much stronger by exercising in the high end of the heart-healthy range. Seventy-five percent of your pulse limit is a strenuous workout indeed. Go there only if you have a clear reason or specific goal other than your heart's benefit. Don't turn your workouts into burnouts.

Figure 15.1	**PULSE LIMIT — MALE**			
Age Group	**Pulse Limit**	55% of Pulse Limit	60% of Pulse Limit	75% of Pulse Limit
20 – 29	**48**	27	29	36
30 – 39	**46**	25	28	34
40 – 49	**43**	24	26	33
50 – 59	**41**	22	25	31
60 – 69	**38**	21	23	29

Pulse rates are for a 15-second time period.

Next to knowing what intensity you should exercise at, you should know how long and how often to do it. Earlier I suggested a minimum guideline of 20 minutes, three times a week. This is an average based on the physical responses and preferences of men and women. To strengthen your heart and vascular system, you need more. How much more depends on your age. If you are in your twenties, thirties, or forties, aerobically exercise at least five days a week. For each age group, however, the length of a workout varies. A man in his twenties should work out at his target rate for 30 minutes; a man in his thirties should work out for 35 minutes; and a man in his forties should work out for 40 minutes. At age 50 or older, you can cut back to 35 minutes. But that's only if you want to. You can, of course, keep your workouts longer, and most people who regularly exercise do.

Moderate aerobic exercise protects your cardiovascular system in another way: it improves stress resilience. But when a big stressor strikes, cut back on your program. Under severe stress, men tend to do just the opposite, almost as if you are trying to burn the bad day or stressor out of your systems. With this response the only thing you burn out is yourself. The stressor is unaffected. No exercise program is written in stone. As with any business, it must be managed under changing conditions.

As the source of so many benefits—more energy, better sleep, uplifted mood—aerobic exercise is an easy product to sell. But its fortification of your heart is the best reason to buy it.

NUTRITION FOR LIVING LONGER

Nutrition is the second most important fitness component for men. In many cases a man's knowledge of nutrition is so poor that his dietary habits can devastate his physical and emotional well-being. Women tend to know more about nutrition. Their ongoing struggle with weight has forced them to gather knowledge. But that doesn't make it any easier for a married executive because his wife cannot give him all the help he needs. She doesn't know, for example, how his vitamin and other nutrient requirements differ from hers. And she doesn't know how to adjust his food intake for increasing amounts of exercise.

Troublesome Red Meat Protein and Fat

A funny thing happens when men start to exercise: they crave protein—steak in particular. Joe, an avid weight lifter since his college days, enjoys telling the story of his first business trip to Texas. He had looked forward to the opportunity for a long time, not only because it represented a career move in his chosen direction, but because he would get to dine at a famous Texas steak house where most of the executives in his company had broken bread. He ordered the biggest steak they had—a 20-ounce monster that even Joe, renowned for his huge appetite, could barely finish. Proud of his feat, Joe was sure he had enhanced his health and his build.

This illogical craving for protein, red meat in particular, continues to ferment in the male consciousness today. The process of building muscles does require more protein, but only a minuscule amount. The average man eats twice as much protein as he should, and as he move up the socioeconomic ladder the imbalance *increases.* Where this leaves the male executive is not good. You must drastically reduce protein, especially red meat, in your diet. Cutting protein confers two important health benefits: it ends the abuse your kidneys take processing excessive protein, and it dramatically lowers your intake of the saturated fat so generously marbling those steaks you long for.

Which brings us to another problem particular to the male executive's diet—too much fat. Way too much. Again, part of this problem stems from the false association of meat protein with strength and health. But another part is due simply to inattention. It's obvious that a pat of butter is fatty. Not so obvious are many other fat traps you can slide into. Take the meal Frank arranged for his clients at a Japanese steak house. Is there anything outlandishly fatty about Japanese food, much of it rice and vegetables? Not to Frank, who liked the idea of everyone sitting around a grill, enjoying the talent and humor of a Japanese chef as he prepared their meals. Unfortunately, everything—the meat, the vegetables, even the rice—was fried. Any executive trying to avoid fat can slide into that kind of trap. So when you arrange, or influence the arrangements of, business lunches or dinners, consider the fat content of the meals. Always include an option to eat low fat. You'll be doing yourself and everyone else a favor.

"Health Insurance" for Men

Besides eating less fat, you can protect your heart by eating more antioxidants. Better known as vitamin C, vitamin E, and beta-carotene, these substances are found in certain fruits and vegetables, the basis behind health professionals' insistence that you eat at least four servings of each a day. Easier said than eaten. Heart protection requires 500 milligrams of vitamin C, 400–800 International Units (IU) of vitamin E, and at least 20,000 IU of beta-carotene daily. These amounts you can get from produce only if you eat great quantities of it. Men won't do that. What you need is an easy source of antioxidants—in short, vitamin supplements—to create a second line of defense against heart disease.

Another substance men don't get enough of is fiber. Yet in its two forms, soluble and insoluble, it has a special importance to a man. Soluble fiber, the recently deified ingredient of oatmeal and oat bran, protects the heart by lowering your cholesterol level. To get this benefit, however, you need to develop a liking for these foods. It takes at least two servings or one generous bowl of oatmeal or oat bran a day.

Insoluble fiber, found in wheat bran, protects the bowel from cancer and keeps you regular. Get it into your diet via a fiber-rich breakfast cereal, but don't choose a cereal by the boasts on the box—they're designed by marketers, not nutritionists. Read the nutritional label. If you don't want to eat it for breakfast, snack on it instead. Or sprinkle it on a salad or in a sandwich. Mix it with anything you want, but eat it.

One mineral men have no trouble sprinkling is salt. Salt is well loved by men—so well loved that you eat far more of it than women do. Used in moderation, salt poses no health risks. But too much of it worsens high blood pressure, a disease that plagues men much more than women. High blood pressure slowly destroys your body—your heart, your kidneys, your brain. Take steps against it before it develops.

The problem is what steps can you take when most salt in your diet comes not from the salt shaker but from the precooked and processed foods you tend to rely on? First see if there are other brands with less salt. If not, think about cooking those foods with a part potassium salt substitute, which has been shown to decrease blood pressure.

Finally, we arrive at aspirin, the non-nutrient I'll close nutrition with because it's one of the easiest safeguards to take. Small doses of aspirin lessen the likelihood of heart attacks, hence taking it as a supplement is now widely recommended for men. But consult your doctor before taking it regularly. If you have no special health problems that preclude it, you will no doubt get the go-ahead. Many male doctors take it themselves.

Male executives tend to be more inflexible than female executives are about their diets. For many years the ability to eat more without gaining weight and to hide what weight they did gain better—especially in a business suit—allowed bad eating habits to flourish. But you weren't getting away with anything, and the heart disease statistics prove it. As a business leader and example for others, turn those statistics around by striving for a healthy body inside as well as outside. Begin by educating yourself about nutrition. Read labels on the food you buy. Read low-fat cookbooks. Read articles from reputable journals. Experiment with new foods and commit yourself to changing. Thus far you have led the way by maintaining reasonable body weights. Now you must step forward again for a healthier diet and longer life.

MAN-AGING STRESS

Have you ever wondered why certain high-potency multivitamins are advertised as "stress" formulas? The rationale lies in the link between stress and heart disease. If a vitamin, specifically one containing antioxidants, can protect the heart, one of the favorite targets of stress, it must be able to protect against stress in general. This is marketing nonsense. No pill, vitamin or otherwise, counters stress. What counters stress is stress resilience.

Although almost anyone in today's society can probably benefit from stress resilience, no group needs it more than male executives. The reason is their Type-A personality. In no other group is Type-A personality more prevalent; it is literally a vehicle to success. Most men realize this and, indeed, are proud of it. A superficial look at the matter tells you why. Hardworking, perfectionistic, efficiency-minded, loyal, conscientious, competitive, and aggressive are all descriptive words found in the definition of this personality, but the most important description is successful. Unfortunately, "success" in these terms is paid for dearly with your health.

Yet you wouldn't want to junk this vehicle—it has taken you too far. Instead, repair it. For male executives this is a matter of life and death because their personality traits are felt to be responsible for the heart disease that ends the careers of so many men just as they enter their prime. Therefore, remove the aggressiveness and competitiveness so the vehicle can run smoothly—without backfiring the black cloud of hostility these traits arouse.

Men do business in an aggressive, competitive way. On the surface it may seem like a productive approach. But inside your body a different plot unfolds. Aggressiveness and competitiveness induce an unhealthy hormonal pattern that leads to emotional tension, a suppressed immune system, high blood sugar, and high blood pressure. Mere nuisances, some executives will say—not worth worrying about when you consider the success that good old-fashioned competition buys. Well it is worth worrying about. What is bad for your body is bad for your mind. If you think that doesn't affect your performance, consider this: hostility stifles your creativity and ability to reason—it actually robs you of business success.

While a female executive has the Type-A characteristics just described, her aggressive and competitive tendencies are minor compared with those of her male counterpart. She has other concerns. As a male, you must internalize your competitiveness—be your best instead of better than someone else. Recognize and mute the aggressive and hostile tendencies when they surface; they're getting you nowhere.

Men can also improve their stress resilience by being more open with others. Many successful executives learned early in their careers to build a foundation of support from their mentors, peers, and subordinates. But this is support on a business and professional level. Support on a personal level—your family and friends— requires a different kind of openness. When you have a problem or even an impending problem, discuss it with your spouse or a friend. Unlike crying or complaining, a calm discussion with a caring person diffuses the impact of problems by confirming the love and support behind you. Bottling up problems inside you isn't a sign of strength; it's a sign of weakness, and it will weaken your stress resilience.

And this weakness makes turning to alcohol very easy during stressful situations. Alcohol interferes with both your mental and motor function. It prevents you from solving a problem by dulling your logical reasoning and your creativity, and it disrupts your sleep at a time when you need it most. Men are more vulnerable to alcoholism than women; they don't even need a family history to harbor the tendency for a "quick fix." Their "cure," however, can turn into a far greater problem than the one they were trying to anesthetize.

FLEX YOUR FLEXIBILITY

Muscular fitness is the last component of a man's program. Literally and figuratively this is a strength in men; in fact it's such a strength that men tend to take it for granted and ignore its ally, flexibility. Why do men neglect their flexibility? Perhaps it's the same reason your closet is messy or your basement cluttered or your garage jammed with junk. It's not a high priority in your life. Or you don't know how important it really is. Whatever the reason, you're not taking the time to do anything about it.

One of the reasons men are less flexible than women is simply that they have more muscle and less estrogen. In a program where muscles develop (that should be any fitness program) it's important that they develop correctly. Flexibility promotes proper muscle development. Building muscles without working on flexibility creates a strong but taut muscle, a situation that invites injury. That's the other benefit of flexibility: it prevents injury.

But don't take this to mean that men who exercise are more prone to inflexibility than sedentary men. As you age, you lose your normal range of motion. This alone leaves you vulnerable to injuries. A sedentary man, who generally doesn't move around much, is even more vulnerable, though he rationalizes that the aches, pains, and cracking joints are part of life. None of these complaints is part of life if you stretch. That is the clinical reason to stretch.

There is, however, a more compelling reason to stretch for the male executive: physical presence. A good suit can hide a few pounds and add some muscle, but it will not lend anything to your posture or generate an ease of movement. Neglecting your flexibility contributes to poor posture, which can rob inches from your height. It also makes your movements slow, choppy, and indecisive, forcing you to appear more anxious than you are. No executive needs that. Stretching exercises inject a spontaneity and fluidity into your body language that exudes a relaxed and commanding confidence. More than one career promotion has come down to that.

Chapter 6 (Figure 6.2) illustrates stretches for your entire body. Do them only when your muscles are warm. It shouldn't be hard to find the right time; flexibility exercises, more than any other exercises, fit well at the office. No props or equipment are necessary—only the will to do it and snatches of time throughout the day.

Another aspect of muscular fitness is strength, the ability to lift and move heavy objects without injuring or fatiguing yourself. Unlike women, whose weight-lifting efforts focus on specific parts of their bodies, men usually take a more general approach, working for a muscular look, and they are willing to spend more time and effort than a woman to get it. From decade to decade your emphasis on that look will change only slightly, but the work you must do to maintain it will decrease: the older you get, the easier it is to maintain your strength. But this is a general statement. One part of the body that does require more work as you get older is your abdomen. For that svelte, flat-waisted look, more abdominal exercise is needed to keep the transverse abdominal muscles along your sides strong.

Do not, however, expect any abdominal exercise to burn fat. On a man, the abdomen is the first place fat collects. True, exercise is the prescription here, but it's aerobic exercise of large muscle groups that burns fat all over, not just in one spot.

The mention of aerobic exercise brings our journey full circle. We started with it as a route to heart health. We end with it as a waist trimmer. It's a perfect example of how one component of fitness can enrich your life in different ways. But you won't discover it by just reading this. Design your own fitness program and live it yourself.

SAMPLE EXERCISE PROGRAMS FOR MEN

The exercise routines in Figure 15.2 are divided into age groups which take into account the physiological changes that occur as you get older. For an example of what a daily and weekly program could look like; see Figure 15.3. It shows how a 40-year-old might map out his road to fitness.

Figure 15.2   **EXERCISING BY AGE GROUP (MALE)**

TWENTIES			THIRTIES		

Aerobic

At least 30 minutes/day
5 days per week
60 – 70% of pulse limit

Aerobic

At least 35 minutes/day
5 days per week
65 – 75% of pulse limit

Flexibility

Stretches (Chapter 6, Fig. 6.2)

Flexibility

Stretches (Chapter 6, Fig. 6.2)

Anaerobic	Sets	Reps	**Anaerobic**	Sets	Reps
Shoulders			*Shoulders*		
Side lifts	2–3	Low	Side lifts	1	Med
				1	Low
Front lifts	2–3	Low	Front lifts	1	Med
				1	Low
Chest			*Chest*		
Barbell bench press	1	Low	Barbell bench press	1	Med
				1	Low
Supine flies	1	Med	Supine flies	1	Med
Arms			*Arms*		
Dumbbell curls	2	Low	Dumbbell curls	2	Low
Triceps barbell curls	1	Low	Triceps barbell curls	1	Med
	1	Med		1	Low
Back			*Back*		
Reverse flies	2	Med	Reverse flies	2	Med
One-arm rowing	2	Low	One-arm rowing	1	Low
Legs			*Legs*		
Reverse leg lifts	1	Med	Reverse leg lifts	1	Med
Weighted leg extensions	1	Low	Weighted leg extensions	1	Med
Heel raises	1	Med	Heel raises	1	Med
Abdomen			*Abdomen*		
Sit-ups	2	Max	Sit-ups	2	Max
Optional			*Optional*		
Push-ups	2	Max	Push-ups	2	Max

Low rep   –   Weighted so that only 3 to 8 repetitions are possible.
Med rep   –   Weighted so that only 10 to 15 repetitions are possible.
High rep   –   Weighted so that 15 to 25 repetitions are possible.
Max   –   As many sit-ups and push-ups as possible.

Figure 15.2 (continued).

FORTIES			FIFTIES and UP		

Aerobic

At least 40 minutes/day
5 days per week
65 – 70% of pulse limit

Aerobic

At least 35 minutes/day
4 or 5 days per week
60 – 70% of pulse limit

Flexibility

Stretches (Chapter 6, Fig. 6.2)

Flexibility

Stretches (Chapter 6, Fig. 6.2)

Anaerobic	Sets	Reps	Anaerobic	Sets	Reps
Shoulders			*Shoulders*		
Side lifts	1	Med	Side lifts	2	Med
	1	Low			
Front lifts	2	Med	Front lifts	1	Med
Chest			*Chest*		
Barbell bench press	1	Low	Barbell bench press	1	Med
Supine flies	1	Med	Supine flies	1	Med
Arms			*Arms*		
Dumbbell curls	1	Med	Dumbbell curls	1	Med
	1	Low			
Triceps barbell curls	2	Med	Triceps barbell curls	1	Med
Back			*Back*		
Reverse flies	2	Med	Reverse flies	1	Med
One-arm rowing	1	Low	One-arm rowing	1	Med
Legs			*Legs*		
Reverse leg lifts	1	High	Reverse leg lifts	1	High
Weighted leg extensions	1	Med	Weighted leg extensions	1	Med
Heel raises	1	Med	Heel raises	1	Med
Abdomen			*Abdomen*		
Sit-ups	2	Max	Sit-ups	1	Max
Reverse trunk twists	2	Med	Reverse trunk twists	2	Med
Optional			*Optional*		
Push-ups	2	Max	Push-ups	2	Max

Low rep	–	Weighted so that only 3 to 8 repetitions are possible.
Med rep	–	Weighted so that only 10 to 15 repetitions are possible.
High rep	–	Weighted so that 15 to 25 repetitions are possible.
Max	–	As many sit-ups and push-ups as possible.

Figure 15.3   **SCHEDULE FOR 40-YEAR-OLD MALE**

WEEKLY	A.M.	P.M.
MONDAY	Aerobic – 40 minutes – 65% pulse limit	Weight lifting – Shoulders – Arms – Legs (optional) – Abdomen
TUESDAY	Aerobic – 40 minutes – 70% pulse limit	Weight lifting – Back – Chest – Abdomen
WEDNESDAY	Aerobic – 40 minutes – 65% pulse limit	Weight lifting – Shoulders – Arms – Legs (optional) – Abdomen
THURSDAY	Aerobic – 40 minutes – 70% pulse limit	Weight lifting – Back – Chest – Abdomen
FRIDAY	Aerobic – 40 minutes – 65% pulse limit	Weight lifting – Shoulders – Arms – Legs (optional) – Abdomen
SATURDAY	Aerobic – Optional – Low or high intensity	Weight lifting – Back – Chest – Abdomen

DAILY	
A.M.	**Warm-up:** 5 minutes slow aerobic **Aerobic:** 40 minutes at heart rate of 117 for a little over 4 miles **Cool-down:** slow aerobic for 3 minutes **Stretches:** from Chapter 6, Fig. 6.2 for 6 minutes
LUNCH	**Stretching:** 5 minutes upper or lower body **Stress Management:** progressive relaxation, meditation, imagery **Weight Lifting:** all or part of P.M. routine (if gym available) **Aerobic:** all or at least 20 minutes of A.M. workout or cross-training
P.M.	**Warm-up:** general total body warm-up before weight lifting,sit-ups are excellent for that, then before each exercise briefly go through the motions with a light weight **Weight Lifting:** Shoulders — side lifts, front lifts, push-ups Arms — dumbbell curls, triceps barbell curls Legs — reverse leg lifts, weighted leg ext., toe raises Abdomen — Sit-ups **Stretching and Cool-down:** 5 minutes upper body stretch

CHAPTER 16

A WOMAN'S PROGRAM

Women are not small men. Strong cultural influences and physical differences including the brain's development in a contrasting hormonal environment all make women different. Even when raised under the same conditions as a man, a woman would still mature with different needs and concerns. Women need a fitness program based not on what's been proposed in the past—that is most assuredly geared for the "weaker sex"—but a program that acknowledges their true potential. In your busy life as both an executive, whose career demands extensive time commitments, and a homemaker, whose skills are indispensable in running a household, it is easy to forget your own needs. To others, the time and energy you invest in your fitness program appears to be for you. But, ultimately, everyone benefits. Airlines always advise parents to put their oxygen masks on first before attending to their children. It's sound advice that fits your entire life—take care of yourself, and you will be better able to take care of your career and your family.

First discussed in a woman's program is aerobic exercise, followed by muscular fitness, stress resilience and attitude, and nutrition, an order based on the probable importance to a woman. Consider it a flexible guide. For you a component other than aerobic exercise might need attention first—perhaps you already run and feel weight lifting is your next priority. Whatever component you start with, it should be the one most lacking in your life.

LIGHT AEROBIC EXERCISE BURNS FAT

In the business world today, the competitive edge can be anything from a chemical formula to the market timing. Often it has to do with the look of a product. Clothing, hotels, restaurants, automobiles, even eyewear, rely to a great extent on appearances. As an executive, the product you offer the marketplace is your technical knowledge, creativity, and ability to manage people as well as corporate resources. Does this have anything to do with appearance? Yes. An executive's performance, appraised objectively, may in theory have nothing to do with how she looks, but total objectivity is impossible with humans, as our attitudes and prejudices unconsciously act on our evaluations. You might say that's unfair. But it's a fact.

Who looks more professional, the overweight, out-of-shape executive, or the trim, fit one? The answer of course is the latter. A fit executive looks more the part, and her condition demonstrates the ability to control one of the hardest areas of her life, her weight. It's an outer look that reflects an inner confidence. Being able to control your weight, you actually feel more confident, better able to handle life's relentless demands after having already jumped one of the highest hurdles.

Does this same rule apply to a man's appearance? To a lesser degree it does, though one man's sloppy, overweight appearance is his fellow staffer's edge toward the promotion they both seek. But men have an easier time than women do controlling their weight, and they can get away with a few extra pounds. Not that women are weaker in the face of food—women tend to be better informed and more disciplined about it than men. It's your physiology that makes it easier for you to put on weight. Before menopause, a woman's hormones protect her from cardiovascular disease. That's the good news. The bad news, however, is that these same hormones are responsible for depositing fat on certain parts of your anatomy and for making it much more difficult to remove that fat.

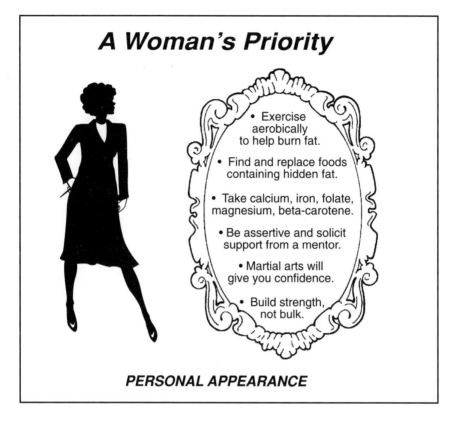

A Woman's Priority

- Exercise aerobically to help burn fat.
- Find and replace foods containing hidden fat.
- Take calcium, iron, folate, magnesium, beta-carotene.
- Be assertive and solicit support from a mentor.
- Martial arts will give you confidence.
- Build strength, not bulk.

PERSONAL APPEARANCE

This, in the presence of a strong cultural bias toward a slimmer woman, presents a problem to every professional, and nine times out of ten, the solution to this problem is aerobic exercise.

To benefit your cardiovascular system, you should exercise three times a week, for 20 minutes at a time, between 60 and 75 percent of your pulse limit (see Figure 16.1). It's a fairly rigorous workout, especially above 70 percent. It's also a typically masculine approach; women younger than 50 don't have to exercise this hard. At a mild intensity, between 50 to 60 percent of your pulse limit, you burn fat—exactly what you want to get rid of. Increase that intensity and you burn progressively more stored carbohydrates and less fat. If weight control is your goal, a less intense workout is your mode. And as research has shown, you are far more likely to stick to a lighter exercise regimen than you are to an intense one. The macho approach doesn't work. Nor should it.

Figure 16.1   **PULSE LIMIT — FEMALE**

Age Group	Pulse Limit	Beginner 45% of Pulse Limit	Fat Burning 55% of Pulse Limit	Cardio 60% of Pulse Limit
20 – 29	48	22	27	29
30 – 39	46	21	25	28
40 – 49	43	20	24	26
50 – 59	41	18	22	25
60 – 69	38	17	21	23

Pulse rates are for a 15-second time period.

Aerobic exercise also addresses another fact of a female executive's life: that she is subjected to substantially more stressors than a male executive. Some are externally generated by the additional demands she must shoulder to climb the corporate ladder. Others are internally generated by her own expectations and the demands she makes on herself. Together they create a high-stress existence. Under such a circumstance, a strenuous workout becomes a stressor itself—just what a woman doesn't need. What a woman does need is a *moderate* workout; moderate aerobic exercise is her protection in an environment where the stress won't let up.

Control over your weight and better stress resilience and the greater self-esteem that both these changes promote are powerful feedback that makes exercise a valued routine used to shake off the negatives of the day. How much exercise is needed to get this feedback depends on your age. If you are in your twenties, exercise at a lighter intensity of 55 percent of your pulse limit for about 35 minutes at a time, five days a week. In your thirties, adjust this regimen slightly by turning up the intensity to 57 percent for 40 minutes, five days a week. Notice you're still below the heart-healthy intensity but getting closer to it. In your forties you reach it. At this age, exercise at 60 percent of your pulse limit for 40 minutes a day to prepare yourself for one of life's biggest transitions, menopause. Menopause changes a woman's hormonal balances. No longer will estrogen shield you from cardiovascular disease, and you must compensate with another kind of protection. Therefore a woman over 50 should exercise above 60 percent of her pulse limit. The increase in intensity comes with a break: you can cut back on your exercise time, keeping your heart rate at its target pulse for only 35 minutes. Thirty-five minutes. Considering the protection you're getting, that's not much time.

It is, however, too much time for any beginner. All the preceding age-related workouts are eventual points to work up to. No one in her forties or fifties, or twenties for that matter, should start an exercise program by working out aerobically 35 minutes a day. Perhaps you consider yourself already active. But if what keeps you active isn't your chosen aerobic exercise, it counts for little. If you are new to an exercise, start gradually: follow the 10 percent rule for time and intensity and listen to your body.

Only after you have developed a solid exercise habit and adequately conditioned your muscles should you reach your recommended workout. Consider it an accomplishment but not necessarily an end point. If you crave a challenge, by all means lengthen your workout or push your heart higher. You'll end up fitter and able to eat more without gaining weight—perhaps the most powerful incentive to exercise aerobically.

BODY SHAPING

Strength is a rare commodity to many women who are conditioned to think that weak muscles are normal. They're not normal. What they are is an insult to a woman's potential.

Here again we wrestle with a cultural bias that has pounded into many heads that women, hampered by some built-in biological handicap, shouldn't get strong and that those who do get strong do it at the risk of their health and sexuality. Yet women need strength as much as men—perhaps more. Today doctors, trainers, and physical therapists advise women to build strength. I purposefully avoided the phrase build your body, complete with its connotations of bulging muscles, because women don't develop big muscles. Your hormones and genetic makeup won't allow it. So what explains those bulging, greased women you may have seen on magazine covers? Extraordinary workouts, with perhaps some help from steroids. No woman needs such a workout and no man does either.

Build Strength Selectively

To build strength, exercise anaerobically. More commonly known as weight lifting or resistance exercise, this is also the best exercise for firming flabby areas of the body. There is no such thing as spot reducing. Exercising specific muscles doesn't chew up the fat around them. But strengthening muscles, which *slightly* expands them, will firm flab by stretching the layer of fat so it's not as noticeable.

Where you focus your weight lifting—arms, chest, back, lower body—depends on your goals, but first strengthen your entire upper body. Most women are frightfully weak there. Then as you get older, focus on specific areas. Women in their twenties and early thirties, for example, generally want well-formed shoulders, front arms (biceps), and legs. As women move into their late thirties and early forties, the emphasis switches to their abdomens and back arms (triceps). Later in their forties and beyond, breast form and support becomes foremost. Always keep in mind, however, that balance is important. Too much energy devoted to one particular area will create an imbalance, and that can lead to injury.

Focus not only delivers more dramatic change to what you consider a problem spot on your body, it also adds motivation to your weight lifting by giving you a goal. Often the goal is a certain look. But that's not the only factor that should motivate you; the increase in strength itself pays other dividends. The last thing a female executive wants is the appearance that she is weak, incapable, and willing to wait for a man to do something that requires any strength. Your resourcefulness in strength-requiring tasks will be admired and appreciated by your male peers and superiors.

From this discussion on strength building you might think it's primarily an upper body activity; it isn't. Resistance exercises also improve your lower body. Many women—and men for that matter—think these are unnecessary. They think their aerobic exercises, which do exercise the lower body, should suffice. But sometimes extra lower body strength is needed. If you want better leg definition, build your calf muscles with resistance exercises. If you want to protect your knees, build your quadriceps.

Women are more prone to chronic knee problems than men are. The reason: men have stronger muscles around their knees. Weak muscles combined with an off-center knee cap is a recipe for pain and even swelling when a woman takes part in high-impact exercises, walks down stairs, or just stands after being seated for a long time. Fortunately, the cure for most cases isn't drugs or surgery; it's exercise. By strengthening the inside of the thigh muscles, the sufferer can stop the painful shifting and grinding of her knee cap.

If this sounds like a hard sell of resistance exercise for women, it is. Resistance exercise is something all women should do because so many consume far less calcium than they need. Low calcium intake creates porous and fragile bones. Adding age and hormonal changes to this plight makes it even worse, and women know it. In recent years you have been bombarded with warnings to bolster your bone density. But many of these warnings have been aimed at increasing calcium intake. Few women know they must also do resistance exercises.

The younger you start weight lifting, the stronger your bones will be by the time you reach menopause. Continued weight lifting after menopause helps to keep your bones dense, preventing the onset of osteoporosis, the dread disease that deteriorates bones, leaving them easy to fracture in later life.

I've discussed the reasons you should weight lift, but I haven't discussed why you would enjoy it. For most women weight lifting is entirely new and exciting because of the distinct changes it brings. The absence of flab, the smoothly contoured muscles, the vibrant feeling of being strong, all keep its enjoyment fresh; it's hard not to enjoy seeing and feeling such progress. And weight lifting can be a social activity too. Done at a gym, you can meet exercisers with a variety of backgrounds, some of them staunch weight lifters and some of them cross-trainers, building strength to improve their performance in other sports. Not that weight lifting at home has to be a solitary activity. One woman began weight lifting at home to become closer to her weight-lifter son, but nowadays she doesn't mind doing it alone.

As you become stronger, you develop confidence in your strength. Linda, the vice president of a medical search firm, is also an officer in the Army Reserve Nursing Corps, who at 5 feet, 6 inches tall and only 120 pounds, never allows a male soldier to carry her duffel bag for her. It weighs over 60 pounds. She credits regular weight training for her strength and loves the advantages it gives her. Being able to carry her duffel bag around or haul herself into a personnel carrier dressed in full gear is not just a convenience for Linda; it distinguishes her as having the proactive attitude of a leader. That sense of confidence has also left its mark on her civilian career.

The Enjoyment of Stretching

The last aspect of muscular fitness is flexibility. Women's hormones preserve flexibility. What that means is that you are naturally more flexible than men. It doesn't mean that you are naturally flexible enough. All women need to stretch—especially after menopause when hormonal changes put you on the same inflexible plane as a man.

Flexibility is contrary to the rule that allows you to maintain muscle condition by doing less as you get older; in this area age means more. But you won't mind doing it because stretching feels so good.

Chapter 6 (Figure 6.2) illustrates stretches for your entire body. Do them only when your muscles are warm. Make it a favorite pastime. Stretching the body is like stretching the mind; you feel as if you can go anywhere and do anything.

PREGNANCY AND EXERCISE

In the past, many doctors have steered pregnant women away from exercise, feeling that it was safer for their patients to forgo it. Times have changed. The latest research shows that women who exercised regularly throughout their pregnancy had healthy babies that were heavier than the babies of women who didn't exercise—proof that exercise benefits the fetus. Still, exercising during pregnancy is not to be taken lightly. It demands an even more attentive approach. (See Figure 16.2.)

During an uncomplicated pregnancy, some exercise is always better than none. But "some exercise" doesn't mean just any pulse raising activity; for whatever you do, you must be properly conditioned. Never begin or intensify an exercise regimen during pregnancy. To safely bike ride, for example, you should have been doing it regularly at least four months before conception. This

Figure 16.2	**PREGNANCY AND EXERCISE**

Cardio	Yes	No
	Swimming	Rowing
	Stairclimbing	Cross-country skiing *
	Cycling	Rope jumping
	Walking	Martial arts
	Running	Recumbant bike
	Aerobics	Exercise (lying on back)

Intensity	– Stay under 70% of pulse limit or heart rate of 140.
Body temp.	– Do not exceed 101 degrees Fahrenheit.
Duration	– Depends on experience and body temperature.
Fluids	– Drink 10 oz of water (or sports drink) every half hour starting 1 hour before and ending 1 hour after workout.
Warm-up	– Perform your chosen exercise at a mild intensity for 5 minutes; then taper up to your regular intensity over another 5 minutes (total of 10 minutes).
Cool-down	– Taper your intensity down for 5 minutes.
Final weeks	– Taper your exercise down during the final 6 weeks of pregnancy by decreasing the intensity and exercising for no more than 25 minutes at a time.

* Cross-country skiing is acceptable if you don't lean on the hip rest with your abdomen.

Muscular

Do not use weights that can only be lifted 3 to 10 times.

Lift relatively light weights doing between 10 and 25 repetitions.

Do not change from a machine routine to a free-weight routine.

Consider changing from a free-weight routine to a machine routine.

Do not do sit-ups in the last two trimesters. Strong abs are great for pregnant women — they save the back and are helpful during delivery — but work on them before pregnancy.

Maintain stretching routine but don't stretch to the point of mild discomfort. Stretch to a point where you've been able to stretch before and where you can feel the muscle stretch.

Precautions

No saunas, hot tubs, or jacuzzis.

Do not initiate a new program or intensify an existing one after becoming pregnant.

advice is especially important if you want to do an impact exercise. Impact exercises—walking, running, aerobic dance—stress bones and joints. It's a positive stress that ultimately leads to stronger bones and joints. During pregnancy, however, your body can't adapt to this stress: the calcium needed to reform bones into stronger, more impact resistant structures, is not available, and the connective tissue, which has become more elastic, cannot give your joints the stability they need.

Assuming that you're already properly conditioned for an impact exercise, the final decision to do it depends on your comfort. Many pregnant women find impact exercises uncomfortable. If you do, switch to a nonimpact cross-training exercise like cycling, stairclimbing or cross-country skiing.

It's always better to go into a pregnancy well trained, but you may not be able to continue the exercise that got you that way. Any exercise that traumatizes or squeezes the abdomen is off limits. Such is the case with rowing; beyond a certain point in your pregnancy its motion will squeeze your abdomen. So will using the arm attachment and pelvic stabilizer of a cross-country ski machine. But unlike rowing, cross-country skiing can be modified into an exercise that's safe to do. Instead of using the arm attachment, steady yourself by holding the handles most models have and keep your abdomen away from the pelvic stabilizer. The only other activity that is absolutely forbidden during pregnancy is martial arts. Women have much to gain from martial arts. But at this time the risks outweigh the gains.

One exercise that gains merit in the maternity world is swimming. Swimming has no impact, but even more important, its water environment keeps your body temperature down. For a pregnant woman, body temperature is a crucial factor in controlling exercise intensity. A body temperature above 101 degrees Fahrenheit can damage the fetus. If you wish to exercise with a fair intensity— assuming that your pregnancy is uncomplicated and that you've had a long established regimen of such workouts—keep your surroundings cool, either with air conditioning or a fan. Above all, drink plenty of fluids. Proper hydration is pivotal in preventing overheating. From one hour before exercising until one hour after you're finished, drink 10 ounces of fluids every 30 minutes. And if you're exercising outdoors, wear layers so that you can remove them as you heat up.

In my discussion of aerobic exercise (Chapter 5), I use heart rate as the gauge of exercise intensity, and even though your body temperature *must* be watched, heart rate remains a good way to monitor your workout. The maximum heart rate a pregnant woman should have during exercise is 140 beats per minute. Compared to my recommendation of 55 to 60 percent of your pulse limit, this may sound high. But a woman's heart rate increases during pregnancy. Factor this natural increase into the rate of 140, and you are still well below the exercise intensity recommended by the American College of Obstetricians and Gynecologists.

None of this is meant to encourage you to exercise intensively while pregnant. Female executives lead high stress lives; you have very demanding jobs and shoulder the lion's share of the household chores. That qualifies as a complication. Therefore, stick with moderate to light workouts. Save the high-intensity ones for the rest of your life.

Pregnancy also affects your warm-up and cool-down routine. A sudden plunge into exercise can divert the blood supply from the fetus to your exercising muscles. To avoid this unhealthy response, warm up 5 minutes longer, taking a total of 10 minutes to gradually increase the intensity of your aerobic exercise to its normal level.

Cooling-down also becomes more important during pregnancy. Never abruptly stop exercising because it can cause a sudden drop in blood pressure. From this anyone can faint, but if you're pregnant the stakes are higher. The sudden drop in blood pressure also reduces blood flow to the fetus. Before you stop exercising, slowly wind down over 5 minutes. At no other time is the gradual approach more important.

Between the warm-up and cool-down is the workout itself. How long should it be? Here there is no pat answer—though obviously this is not the time to increase its duration. Again base your decision on what you're already used to. If your pre-pregnancy workouts lasted 35 minutes, that's a safe amount of time during your pregnancy—unless your temperature tells you otherwise. The longer you exercise, the higher your body temperature gets.

Another time-related question is how far into your pregnancy should you exercise? A survey of women noted that most decreased the intensity and duration of their workouts by the time they delivered. The reason: comfort. My advice is to taper to mild exercise and limit the time to 20 or 25 minutes the last six weeks before delivery. If you run, for example, walk instead.

Not yet discussed in this section is weight lifting. If aerobic exercise used to be frowned upon, anaerobic exercise or weight lifting was outright forbidden—but back then women who weren't pregnant shouldn't have been weight lifting either. All women should weight lift, and as with their aerobic programs, they should continue to do it into their pregnancy. Observe the same exercise guidelines: don't intensify or extend workouts, and as your pregnancy progresses become more conservative. Beyond the first trimester, limit the weight of what you can lift to at least 15 to 20 times. If you work with a weight machine, stay with it; don't start dabbling with free weights. For pregnant women especially, machines are a better alternative. The hormonal changes of pregnancy make the joints less stable. Machines give you more stability, preventing the strains that can happen more easily at this time, and they lessen the likelihood of a mishap involving the abdomen. But during the last six weeks, cease all weight lifting, machine or not. You'll appreciate the rest.

As for stretching, that too belongs in your pregnancy fitness program. Just stay with the status quo. Do not try to stretch your limits.

Exercise is a vital ingredient of everyone's life. When you're pregnant, though certain limitations apply, it becomes more important—you're doing it for two people instead of one.

Overcoming a Woman's Vulnerabilities

Today's female executive must resolve the ultimate conflict, the pull between the dual roles of professional and homemaker. Add motherhood to this scenario and the conflict worsens. Much of the problem stems from the division of labor at home, the woman shouldering 65 percent of the child care and household chores, while the father helps with less than 20 percent. Your job as a professional carries many responsibilities. So does your job as homemaker. Yet you feel you must handle both areas with the same competence you would handle one. This is the curse of "having it all." Brainwashed by the media, you feel you must accomplish an impossible task and out of this dilemma grows tremendous confusion, guilt, and resentment. Supermom just doesn't exist.

No woman can continuously carry such a heavy burden. Yet day after day millions of women keep trying, and the effect on their health is telling. What women caught in this trap need is a break. But this "break" must come from within themselves.

The techniques and suggestions offered in Chapter 14 on stress management are particularly effective for the executive in conflict. So too is regular exercise—it forges much mental and physical resilience. There is, however, a discipline that can generate a more positive attitude and fortify stress resilience while delivering a work-out rich in both strengthening and aerobic exercise. These are the martial arts.

The Martial Arts Offer a Calm Confidence

The martial arts have long had the reputation as a form of violence. Nothing could be further from the truth. The martial arts can be more accurately described as a mental and physical approach to inner peace. One variety called Tai Chi Chuan was said to have been developed for infirm monks so that their bodies "could be a more secure temple for the soul." Another form called Aikido designates one of a practicing pair an Oke. The Oke plays the aggressor, but translated the word means "he who attacks falls."

Any type you choose is likely to offer a complete package, improving your strength, aerobic capacity, balance, and flexibility while fostering a confidence and peacefulness that has been described as an attitude of meditation. You'll also be able to defend yourself.

Claire works at a large municipal hospital. As the administrative assistant to the chairman of the Psychiatric Department, one of her duties was to accompany him on weekly rounds of four psychiatric wards. This, Claire didn't feel, a Masters in Business Administration had prepared her for, and though she had great compassion for the patients on these wards, she was also afraid of them. In fact so afraid was she, that she decided to take karate lessons. Claire found the lessons invigorating, and after eight months she noticed that she felt calm and secure during ward rounds, an attitude that had more to do with the entire discipline of Martial arts than her ability to defend herself. Claire took lessons from a reputable master. Before you register for a class, check out the credentials of the instructor. Then enroll your children too.

Take a Page Out of a Man's Book

Still another way to handle stress is to be assertive. Women, far more than men, are able to discuss personal problems with their family and friends, which is good. But when the stressor is work related, family and friends may not be the best people to turn to. Instead, discuss the problem with someone senior to yourself whom you feel would understand your situation and be able to advise you. Talking to a female mentor might be more comfortable for you, but in today's corporate world, she is not that easy to find. The lack of female mentors has been cited as the most common reason for why a woman's career in both business and the sciences lag behind her male counterpart. You need supportive information. Gender should not matter.

So find a mentor and ask questions. This requires you to be more assertive, something our culture doesn't usually program into your upbringing because it is typically viewed as a male trait. View it as a healthy trait instead. By adopting it, you rid yourself of those feelings of helplessness that lead to anxiety and depression, two states that commonly sap a woman's effectiveness and productivity.

This approach also decreases your tendency to become emotional. Fostered in women since childhood, emotionalism, especially the show of anger, sadness, and outrage, is another behavior that can damage your career. Some kinds of psychotherapy build on the pretense that emotionalism clears the air, thereby refreshing your psyche. It does not. It burns bridges, alienates others, and destroys your inner peace. Discard this so-called feminine feature by substituting it with a demonstration of stability and control. Emotionalism is just another recipe for anxiety and depression.

Unfortunately, to this recipe, a female executive often adds a generous measure of unreasonably high standards and attention to detail. Both are positive characteristics when time is plentiful, but tormentors when time is short (as it so often is for executives), demanding what is, under the circumstances, impossible. No executive needs a rigid approach like this. Free yourself by taking a page out of a man's book: relax your standards, delegate and take shortcuts.

Nutrition for Your Health and Hormones

If women have been cursed, it is with eating. Yet the female executive can least afford to be overweight. For her it is not a matter of vanity, it is a matter of which direction she would like her career to go in.

Part of the curse has to do with your body. Women's bodies store fat more efficiently than men's. If it is not immediately used for energy, it's layered onto your hips. Once stored, fat seems to develop its own instinct for survival, tenaciously clinging to you no matter how little you eat. But really it's not the fat clinging to you. It's your body holding on to it—much more tightly than a man's does.

That solves the mystery of why men lose weight more easily than women. It's not that they know more or have a better diet than women. In fact, you, because of your long war against pounds, know more about food than men do. You know, for example, that one of the keys to weight control is limiting fat in your diet. But woman does not live on knowledge alone. About 50 percent of the average American's calories come from fat, and it's not just men's fatty diets skewing this miserable statistic. Women also eat too much fatty food. The answer to nutritional fitness and permanent weight control is not another "give-up-everything-you-love-to-eat" diet; it's the three-step OptimEating plan in Chapter 13 that is designed to reward you with your favorite foods.

But a woman's eating strategy should go beyond weight control. Vitamins and minerals are important too. Let's start with calcium, the kingpin of your antiosteoporosis campaign. Calcium's Recommended Daily Allowance (RDA) is 800 milligrams (mg) a day, but for women higher doses up to 1500 mg are recommended. The question is: will all this calcium get to your bones? Research indicates it may not without the help of vitamin D. Well, that doesn't seem like a serious problem. Given that vitamin D is in milk and produced by the skin, there would seem to be a plentiful supply of it to do the job. But not all milk is adequately fortified, and even if it were, few women drink as much as it would take to satisfy the requirement. As for the skin, it needs sunlight to produce vitamin D.

Most women don't get much of that during the winter. Therefore, take 400 International Units (IU) of vitamin D a day as extra bone insurance. It's a policy you'll be glad you took out.

Sometimes, however, the best intentions go awry. Here you are taking calcium, taking vitamin D, lifting weights, and what do you reach for at the first sign of thirst—a soft drink. Many soft drinks contain phosphorous. Phosphorous saps your body of calcium. The more soft drinks you drink, the more you downgrade your insurance.

In the body it isn't unusual for one vitamin or mineral to counteract another. Calcium itself can be a counteractor. Taken less than one hour before or less than two hours after a meal, calcium prevents the absorption of iron. Iron is another mineral of specific importance to a woman. Before menopause you lose it regularly during menstruation. Today many women don't consider this a problem. After all, isn't every food fortified with iron? It would seem so. But to eat enough food to satisfy your iron needs, you would have to eat too many calories. In short, eating properly won't give you enough iron. Eat right, but also take a supplement that includes 18 mg of iron.

Iron may not be the only thing your menstrual cycle shorts you on: patience may also be scarce. Although PMS (premenstrual syndrome) is a household term, as well as a psychiatric diagnosis, it is uncommon in the severe form the term actually stands for. What is common are milder symptoms of it. Seven to 12 days before menstruation many women feel tired and out of sorts. Most remedies are prescriptions meant for the severe form of PMS. Unless you are racked that badly, try taking the edge off with 500 mg of magnesium a day one to two weeks before menstruation. For some women this works.

Another supplement needed by women is folate. After a folate deficiency was linked to birth defects, folate became the hot topic of the media, and women of childbearing age were urged to take 400 mg daily—good advice except that it left out a large portion of women who also need the supplement. Folate may prevent or hinder the advance of cervical dysplasia, a precancerous condition of the uterus. Whether you intend to have children or not, this supplement belongs in your diet.

Also in the news lately is the link between diet and breast cancer. Researchers have found that a low-fat, high-fiber diet not only protects against breast cancer; it can slow the spread of the disease.

More protection—and you can never have too much—can come from 20,000 IU daily of beta-carotene. How much protection this will give you is unknown. But a low-fat, high-fiber diet supplemented with beta-carotene is healthy. That's enough reason to take it.

Many women may think that health is a good reason to drink alcohol. According to a highly publicized study, alcohol to some extent prevents the arteries from hardening. What an easy way to protect your heart after menopause has stripped it of its hormonal protection. But alcohol consumption has been linked to breast cancer. Some medical minds think you should weigh the risk by looking at your family history. If you have breast cancer in the family, but no heart disease, avoid alcohol. If you have heart disease in the family, but no breast cancer, one drink a day may not be harmful. God knows what you should do if your family background has both diseases. My advice is to forget alcohol. If you want to avoid heart disease, then eat right and exercise. To advise anyone to drink, in light of all the other health and social problems alcohol causes, is to have absolutely no faith in her ability to take care of her body.

It's unrealistic to expect any woman to eat a diet so stark and disciplined that she could limit her caloric intake while getting all the nutrients she needs. Fill those cracks and crevices in your diet by taking a high-potency multivitamin every day.

When you hear news about some dietary or exercise breakthrough, be skeptical. So much of what's trumpeted by the media is misrepresented in an effort to sensationalize it. Or it's not explained correctly—probably because the writer doesn't understand it. Use your business skills to follow up these claims by checking more reputable sources like health journals or newsletters. Be informed, but be selective of where you get that information. Your diet and exercise regimen are too important to be guided by false claims.

Sample Exercise Programs for Women

The exercise routines in Figure 16.3 are divided into age groups which take into account the physiological changes that occur as you get older. For an example of what a daily and weekly program could look like, see Figure 16.4. It shows how a 40-year-old might map out her road to fitness.

Figure 16.3   *EXERCISING BY AGE GROUP (FEMALE)*

TWENTIES	THIRTIES

Aerobic

At least 35 minutes/day
5 days per week
55% of pulse limit

Aerobic

At least 40 minutes/day
5 days per week
55 – 60% of pulse limit

Flexibility

Stretches (Chapter 6, Fig. 6.2)

Flexibility

Stretches (Chapter 6, Fig. 6.2)

Anaerobic	Sets	Reps	**Anaerobic**	Sets	Reps
Shoulders			*Shoulders*		
Side lifts	2–3	Low	Side lifts	2	Med
Front lifts	2	Low	Front lifts	1	Med
Chest			*Chest*		
Barbell bench press	1	Med	Barbell bench press	1	Med
Arms			*Arms*		
Dumbbell curls	2	Low	Dumbbell curls	1	Low
Triceps barbell curls	1	Med	Triceps barbell curls	2	Low
or kickbacks	1	Med	Kickbacks	2	Med
Back			*Back*		
Reverse flies	1	Med	Reverse flies	1	Med
or one-arm rowing	1	Med	or one-arm rowing	1	Med
Back raises	2	25	Back raises	2	25
Legs			*Legs*		
Reverse leg lifts	1	High	Reverse leg lifts	1	High
Weighted leg extensions	1	Med	Weighted leg extensions	1	Med
Heel raises	2	Med	Heel raises	1	Med
Abdomen			*Abdomen*		
Sit-ups (feet held)	1	Max	Sit-ups (feet held)	1	Max
(feet not held)	1	Max	(feet not held)	1	Max
Optional			*Optional*		
Push-ups			Push-ups		
(not from knees)	1–2	Max	(not from knees)	1–2	Max

Low rep	–	Weighted so that only 3 to 8 repetitions are possible.
Med rep	–	Weighted so that only 10 to 15 repetitions are possible.
High rep	–	Weighted so that 15 to 25 repetitions are possible.
Max	–	As many sit-ups and push-ups as possible.

Figure 16.3 (continued).

| FORTIES | | | FIFTIES and UP | | |

Aerobic

At least 40 minutes/day
5 days per week
60% of pulse limit

Aerobic

At least 35 minutes/day
4 or 5 days per week
60% of pulse limit

Flexibility

Stretches (Chapter 6, Fig. 6.2)

Flexibility

Stretches (Chapter 6, Fig. 6.2)

Anaerobic	Sets	Reps	Anaerobic	Sets	Reps
Shoulders			**Shoulders**		
Side lifts	1	High	Side lifts	1	Med
Front lifts	1	Med	Front lifts	1	Med
Chest			**Chest**		
Barbell bench press	1	Low	Barbell bench press	2	Med
Supine flies	2	Med	Supine flies	2	Med
Arms			**Arms**		
Dumbbell curls	1	Low	Dumbbell curls	1	Med
Triceps barbell curls	2	Med	Triceps barbell curls	1	Med
Kickbacks	2	Med	Kickbacks	1	Med
				1	Low
Back			**Back**		
Reverse flies	2	Med	Reverse flies	1	Med
or one-arm rowing	2	Med	One-arm rowing	1	Med
Back raises	2–3	25	Back raises (weighted)	2	Med
Legs			**Legs**		
Reverse leg lifts	1	Med	Reverse leg lifts	1	Med
Weighted leg extensions	1	Med	Weighted leg extensions	1	Med
Heel raises	1	Med	Heel raises	1	Med
Abdomen			**Abdomen**		
Sit-ups (feet not held)	2	Max	Sit-ups (feet not held)	2	Max
Reverse trunk twists	1	High	Reverse trunk twists	1	High
Optional			**Optional**		
Push-ups	1–2	Max	Push-ups	1–2	Max

Low rep	–	Weighted so that only 3 to 8 repetitions are possible.
Med rep	–	Weighted so that only 10 to 15 repetitions are possible.
High rep	–	Weighted so that 15 to 25 repetitions are possible.
Max	–	As many sit-ups and push-ups as possible.

Figure 16.4   **SCHEDULE FOR 40-YEAR-OLD FEMALE**

WEEKLY	A.M.	P.M.
MONDAY	Aerobic – 40 minutes – 55% pulse limit	Weight lifting – Shoulders – Back – Chest (optional) – Abdomen
TUESDAY	Aerobic – 40 minutes – 60% pulse limit	Weight lifting – Arms – Legs – Abdomen
WEDNESDAY	Aerobic – 40 minutes – 55% pulse limit	Weight lifting – Shoulders – Back – Chest – Abdomen
THURSDAY	Aerobic – 40 minutes – 60% pulse limit	Weight lifting – Arms – Legs – Abdomen
FRIDAY	Aerobic – 40 minutes – 55% pulse limit	Weight lifting – Shoulders – Back – Chest – Abdomen
SATURDAY	Aerobic – Optional	Weight lifting – None

DAILY	
A.M.	**Warm-up:** 5 minutes slow run **Aerobic:** 40 minutes at heart rate of 102 for about 4 miles **Cool-down:** jog for 3 minutes **Stretches:** from Chapter 6, Fig. 6.2 for 5 minutes
LUNCH	**Stretching:** 5 minutes upper body, 5 minutes lower body **Stress Management:** progressive relaxation, meditation, imagery **Weight Lifting:** all or part of P.M. routine (if gym available) **Aerobic:** all or at least 20 minutes of A.M. workout or cross-training
P.M.	**Warm-up:** general total body warm-up before weight lifting, sit-ups are excellent for that, then before each exercise briefly go through the motions with a light weight **Weight Lifting:** Shoulders — side lifts, front lifts, push-ups Back — reverse flies, back raises Chest — barbell bench press, supine flies Abdomen — Sit-ups **Stretching and Cool-down:** 5 minutes upper body stretch

• CHAPTER 17 •

TOTAL FITNESS

Total fitness is an integrated state of body and mind; it is both physical and mental. Physical fitness means a healthy heart and vascular system, strong flexible muscles, and a nutritional status that keeps all systems energized. Mental fitness means a constructive attitude to oversee life's experiences and a stress resilience that is able to deal with the more challenging ones. Together, these components—cardio, muscular, nutrition, attitude, and stress resiliency—build a foundation of excellence that can be yours.

But before you build this foundation, you must understand the components. For clarity and organization, I discussed each component separately. Throughout the book, however, I remind you that the mind and body are really one, and that all components of fitness are one complex interactive mechanism that could only exist in something as marvelous as a human being. For example, aerobic exercise, the kingpin of the cardio component, also improves muscular endurance, nutritional status, stress resilience and attitude. Likewise, changes in nutritional status, stress resilience, and attitude improve the cardiovascular system.

In giving you these examples, I'm not suggesting that there is a linear relationship in how components improve each other. That is an over-simplification and certainly not how the human body works. Improvements in components feed back and forth to each other. When one component gets better, improving a second component, the improved second component then feeds back to the original component, improving it even more. Imagine this going on between five components. It becomes a snowballing effect that not only accrues benefits but compounds them as well.

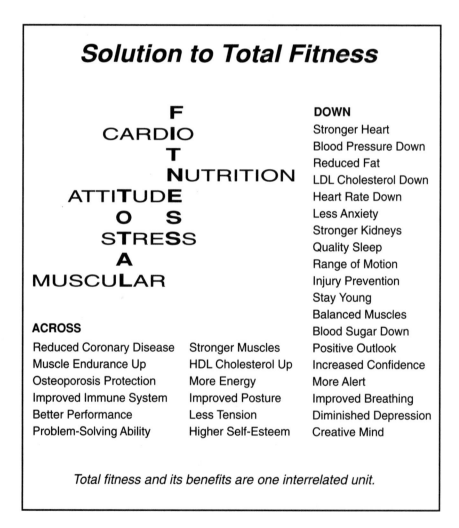

Solution to Total Fitness

```
              F            DOWN
        CARDIO             Stronger Heart
           T               Blood Pressure Down
              NUTRITION    Reduced Fat
                           LDL Cholesterol Down
       ATTITUDE            Heart Rate Down
         O    S            Less Anxiety
                           Stronger Kidneys
        STRESS             Quality Sleep
           A               Range of Motion
    MUSCULAR               Injury Prevention
                           Stay Young
                           Balanced Muscles
```

ACROSS   Blood Sugar Down

Reduced Coronary Disease	Stronger Muscles	Positive Outlook
Muscle Endurance Up	HDL Cholesterol Up	Increased Confidence
Osteoporosis Protection	More Energy	More Alert
Improved Immune System	Improved Posture	Improved Breathing
Better Performance	Less Tension	Diminished Depression
Problem-Solving Ability	Higher Self-Esteem	Creative Mind

Total fitness and its benefits are one interrelated unit.

HOW TO GET STARTED ON YOUR FITNESS LIFESTYLE

A total fitness program of this magnitude cannot be forced into your regular routine. That would make it painful and unwelcome. Yet this is how many executives approach fitness; it is consistent with their management style. They see a significant behavioral change as being the same as a calculated business risk, and they put themselves under incredible pressure to get that change made. It becomes another job. With such good intentions but such a bad approach, what happens to executives next is easy to understand. Caught between the pull of their fitness program and the rest of their responsibilities, they finally yield, giving up their programs for such excuses as time constraints, travel, business crises, or just plain exhaustion. The waves of excuses battering the beaches of their resolve finally erode their programs piece by piece. If this were a product line or a business that failed, they'd analyze the reasons why. But it's a personal fitness program, so they just think it can't be done.

Knowledge of health and exercise is more than a provider of facts. It motivates you to adopt a program of fitness improvements and gives you the information you need to design it. After that you need goals and a gradual approach. The right goals guide and propel you through the process. Short-range goals allow you to partition your progress into recognizable accomplishments. Long-range goals provide direction over a period of months and years. Both support the gradual approach, just the opposite of what executives tend to choose.

In Chapter 1 you answered a fitness questionnaire. Your score is a snapshot of your current physical and emotional condition. Taken by component your score will also tell you where to start—what component of fitness needs the most work. If all your scores are comparable or you're not sure what direction to take, use the order suggested in Chapter 15, "A Man's Program," or Chapter 16, "A Woman's Program." They are based on the average physical and mental fitness of male and female executives. Whatever order you work on the different components of your fitness program, only start on one component at a time.

I won't claim that this orderly approach is immune to roadblocks—the time, the travel, the weather, the injury. But I will say that there will be fewer of them. And when you make fitness a priority, you're certain to invent ways to overcome the roadblocks you do hit, to find the time to exercise, to find a way to exercise on the road. If necessity is the mother of invention, priority is the father. You can find a way. Let that be your motto.

An Executive Couple's Evolving Fitness Program

Three years ago Donna, a clothing buyer for a national retail chain, started walking daily to lose weight. Many people today would say that Donna didn't have a real weight problem. But her business was clothing and lately she was growing out of hers—18 pounds had settled on her 5-foot, 2-inch frame since her college graduation 15 years before. That works out to a little over a pound a year. What would she look like in 10 years? Her response to this realization was to walk at least 30 minutes a day, usually at lunchtime around the parking lot where she worked. She also began to watch the fat content of what she ate and rejoiced when a yogurt stand that sold fatless frozen yogurt opened across the street from her office. Lunch became fatless frozen yogurt. Dinners, previously high-fat meals with her husband and two children, became solo salads with Weight Watchers dressing. It wasn't as radical a change as it seems; Donna drifted into the salad meals gradually. At first they were a sideline to keep her from filling up on the caloric main courses. Then they just got larger and topped with tuna, low-fat cheese, or some "decent leftovers."

About one year later, Donna accompanied her sister-in-law Nancy, a weight lifter, to a women's body-building competition at Madison Square Garden. If Nancy's intention was to get Donna interested in weight lifting, she succeeded. For Christmas, Donna requested and got an inexpensive weight-training machine. There in the basement, leaning against a wall about five feet from the oil burner, it sat—not a very inviting location. But Donna managed to ignore the surroundings and concentrate on weight lifting, using the machine three or four times a week until she accompanied Nancy to a Gold's Gym. This was weight-lifting heaven. Donna now knew what it was like to lift with expensive equipment, and left her Christmas gift to keep the oil burner company.

Meanwhile her husband John, a CPA with his own accounting business, ignored the changes in her eating habits and flatly refused to exercise. This didn't bother Donna, who believed John had a right to choose his own lifestyle—that is, until John's "burrito attack." One evening before leaving for a party, John microwaved two frozen burritos to eat on the way. John was a world-class eater who could finish two dozen chicken wings by himself; a burrito appetizer before a party was not unusual. But that night he didn't get away with it.

On the way to the party, John started having excruciating stomach pains that would continue on and off through the night. They never made it to the party. They did, however, make it to the hospital, where John spent the next four days undergoing tests which led to his having a gall stone removed. Small smooth pebble-like collections of calcium or cholesterol, gall stones are often caused by a fatty diet. For John it was a learning experience—a very painful one. Unless he wanted to go through that pain again, he would have to decrease the fat in his diet, and with Donna's help he did. She no longer makes whole pans of chicken wings for John to eat. Now when she makes them, John gets one serving and the rest are frozen for future dinners. As for those burritos, they're left at the supermarket. If John wants a preparty appetizer, he makes himself a sandwich of diet bread and low-fat cold cuts.

By changing his diet—John was about 30 pounds overweight at the time of the "burrito attack"—he did lose some weight. But not 30 pounds. Still a world-class eater, John managed to hold onto 20 of those pounds through sheer volume eating. The pain hadn't changed his love of food.

Then the ultimatum came. Donna, herself shaken by John's illness, was more aware than ever of his weight problem and his sister Nancy just added fat to the fire. She bluntly informed both John and Donna that he could "drop dead of a heart attack any second." As a social worker in a hospital emergency room, she'd seen it happen. As John's wife, Donna didn't want to see it happen, and she told him that she would never forgive him if he dropped dead on her, so he had better lose weight. Finally, John agreed he should exercise to lose weight. He bought himself a treadmill to run on and he still uses it today.

To look at John and Donna, you would think they've practically got it made: a dual-career couple whose fitness program
evolved with four of the five fitness components—cardio (aerobic
exercise), nutrition, muscular, and attitude (as attitude pertains to
the other three components). But it's not a picture-perfect story. As
you may have noticed, John started exercising for the wrong reason:
Donna's concern. Luckily his half-hearted approach of running only
a mile at a time in the beginning kept him from beating himself up,
and he gradually came to enjoy it, especially after he put a TV in
the basement next to the treadmill. His decision to change his diet
was somewhat better—a way to avoid the worst pain of his life. Yet
both decisions stuck and John's respect for fitness grows each year.

So does Donna's. But unlike John's attitude toward fitness, hers
was correct from the start. She aimed for weight loss and expanded
her program from there. It happened the right way, piece by piece,
starting with a simple campaign of aerobic exercise (walking) and
watching fat in her diet, then moving on to weight lifting at a gym
and more stringent fat-cutting measures (for John). Today Donna
and Nancy regularly put in between 30 and 40 minutes on a stairclimber twice a week. Donna discovered that at the gym too.

Donna and John's story sums up a situation you'll recognize as
you proceed with your fitness program: that it will evolve to fit your
busy life as it continues to improve the quality of it. The longer you
stay with it, the better it gets.

Making It Happen

Roger was known as a tough manager, a reputation he was proud
of. But it was not the tasks he assigned to his engineering staff that
made him tough; it was his reaction to their mistakes and imper-
fections. If someone made an error or submitted a report late, his
reaction would always be anger, raising his voice, making belittling
remarks, beginning every sentence with "damn it." There was no
mistaking the intense displeasure of this 6-foot, 3-inch man.

Still, Roger didn't enjoy "being in a stew," and experience with
certain employees hinted that it wasn't always the most effective
managerial style. Last year his secretary asked for a transfer, and two
out of his staff of six quit. Warned by his boss that such a high

turnover was not a good way to run a department, Roger decided to register for a seminar on motivating employees. It was an uncharacteristic move made for the sake of his career. But the seminar impressed him and he followed it up by doing some of the suggested reading. One authority recommended relaxation exercises as a way to subdue angry reactions to mistakes. He also hoped they would calm the tremor he'd had for six months. His internist, however, had a better idea for that: reduce his coffee intake.

Roger took the advice. If changing his managerial style would make his staff more productive, he would do it. First he relaxed his unreasonable standards. Then, with the help of the relaxation exercises, he started to relax his body and his mind. And he whittled his coffee consumption from 12 to 5 cups a day. It was an impressive effort.

Nevertheless, at times he still got angry, and to Roger these episodes were always a sign of failure. He wondered what it would take to become a truly effective manager. His answer came about a month later. Waiting for a late report, he stood next to his secretary's desk, forcefully tapping his finger on the fax machine. He was fuming and his secretary noticed, remarking that the report must be quite late for him to be that mad. An offhand remark, but it astounded him. This secretary had only worked for him for seven months—she hadn't been subjected to his preseminar tyranny—and she saw him as a different person. Because he *was* a different person. To his secretary, he seemed composed and mild mannered. To the veterans of his staff he seemed like another person entirely. But to himself he seemed like the same person, having made only minor progress.

Roger's mistake was quite common. One reason he failed to recognize his change was that his goal was not specific enough, for example, to decrease the number of angry outbursts from once a week to once a month. But the larger issue here is that of gradual change. Even profound change, when brought about gradually, will seem minor to the person who lives with small increments of it on a daily basis. Such small increments will not draw your attention because they're painless—which happens to be why they last. Yet without obvious proof, you think you've failed, and you give up the program that doesn't seem to work. Don't wait for an offhand remark by someone else to highlight your progress; that comment may never come.

Set specific goals and track your progress toward them. Harness the power of your gradual change by making sure you notice it. If you notice yourself lapsing into old behavior, forgive yourself and go on with your program. Don't let small lapses stand out like failures; they are inevitable—particularly during times of stress. It's a fact of change. But what is also a fact of change is that these lapses are usually a lesser version of the old behavior: Roger's finger tapping used to be his fist slamming. That's a big difference.

Many people go through life reaching goals and never realizing it. They don't step back and look at the big picture, the difference between now and then. This brand of failure is an illusion and any executive will agree that good decisions don't get made with false information.

For your total fitness program to succeed, regularly appraise your current condition, make the right adjustments and form new goals for the future. Use a logbook to write your exercise autobiography and refer to the *PEACE* and *BLISS* cards for guidance in eating and stress resilience. With these tools and a positive, can-do attitude, you will find a way to make total fitness happen to you. After all, making things happen is what successful executives do best. Make it so.

INDEX

303